Fasting the Fat Away:

A Guide to the Intermittent Fasting Diet for Beginners

By:

Linda Becker

Linda Becker

Table of Contents:

Introduction

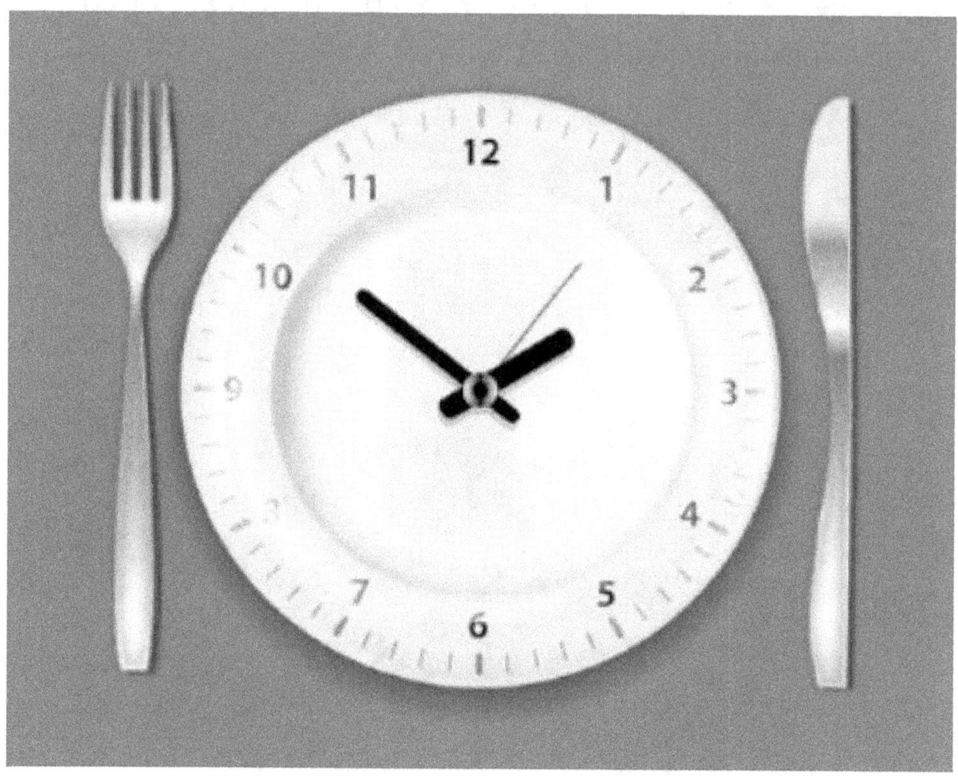

Many thanks for choosing to read this book. Many people today are looking for a diet that works or are seeking ways of eating more healthily. The problem is that there are so many ideas in the bookshops, online and in newspapers and magazines that choosing the right one for you can be a real challenge.

Intermittent fasting not only works in making our bodies healthier, but it also helps with weight loss. This book will offer a detailed insight into intermittent fasting, what it looks like in practice and how to do it. I won't overly simplify it or sugar coat it, but rather present the advantages and challenges alike. People are far more likely to sustain their diet if they are aware from the beginning that sometimes it will be tough.

Of course, while on the one hand it is wise to consider all the options before launching into a change of eating regime; we also have to consider that the longer we procrastinate the harder it is to make a start.

The really good news is that intermittent fasting has moved from the point of being a fad to becoming a widely accepted method of improving the way we eat, and of losing weight. Its popularity comes largely from the combined facts that firstly it works, and secondly it is easy to maintain, and thirdly the science is there.

In many ways this is common sense: by eating fewer meals we are eating fewer calories. If we reduce our calorie intake, we will (almost always) lose weight. Then, intermittent fasting adds nothing to our workload. In fact, it reduces it. By eating two meals a day instead of three, we add nothing to our preparation and cooking time, and save ourselves an hour by taking out a meal.

If the system chosen is to occasionally fast for a day, once again we save ourselves time, and of course money. If breakfast consists of two pastries and a coffee on the way to work, we are going to save ourselves $80 a month from not buying the pastries alone.

In this book we are going to look at all we need to know about this method of ensuring a healthy lifestyle. We will give some background information into the history of intermittent fasting and see it in the context of the cultural situations in which it developed. We will offer a detailed account of the advantages of moving to this kind of lifestyle, but we will also make it clear where it might not be the best option for an individual. We will spend time looking at the scientific reasons behind its success. This will include a look at some of the research, a consideration of its effect on our metabolism, and the benefits these bring.

We will consider the various kinds of fasting, because there are several types. We will also explore the different approaches people take: For example, people can approach intermittent fasting as a form of temporary cleansing, or as a more long-term lifestyle choice.

We will see the explosive affect intermittent fasting can have on your weight loss when appropriately combined with the right kind of exercise to bring about even better health and diet benefits, and we will also look at nutritional factors in using the diet. This will include a consideration of the types of food that work best with intermittent fasting.

I hope you find this information as mind-blowing and

useful as I did.

One: What Is Intermittent Fasting?

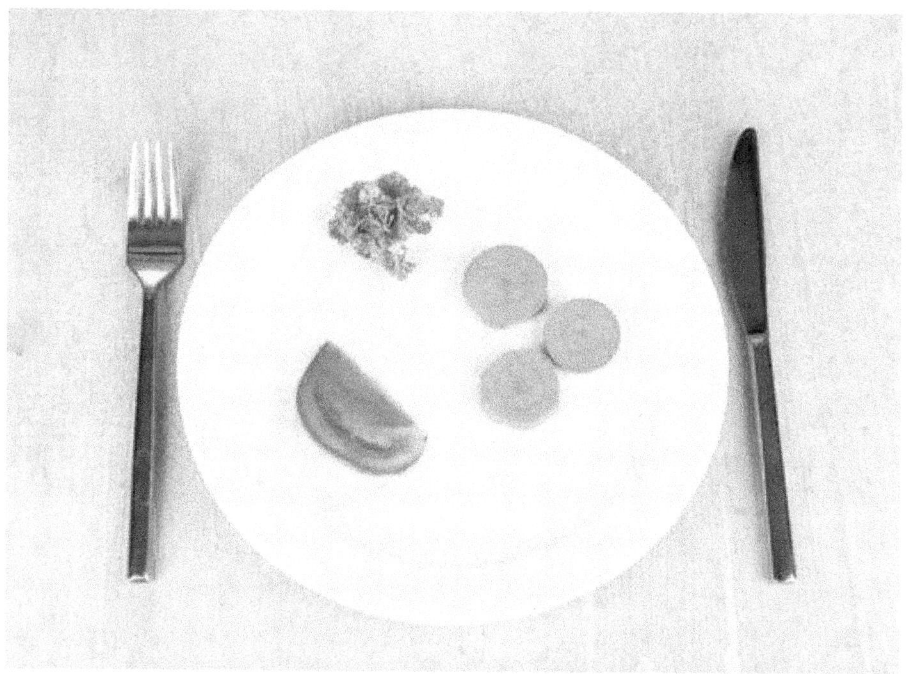

In this chapter, we will look at a clear definition of intermittent fasting. We will also consider some of the myths and misconceptions that exist around the subject. The diet industry is worth billions of dollars worldwide; so, to have something that largely means eating what you want (just not as often) that also delivers excellent results, is a real threat to that industry.

This may be why you hear conflicting messages about intermittent fasting — there are a lot of politics involved and many health and fitness companies will make less money if you discover the amazing secrets of intermittent fasting.

We will consider the history of intermittent fasting, putting it into the context of fasting as a part of various societies' culture. Finally, in this chapter, we will consider those people for whom this is an ideal lifestyle commitment, and those for whom it is less so.

Intermittent Fasting – A Definition

The term literally means occasional fasting, or not eating, during a given period. Broadly, there are two main forms of intermittent fasting. The first of these involves occasional days off from eating. At the more severe end, which would consist of a one-day-eating, one-day-not regime to the more common kind of routine where there is normal eating for six days of the week, and then one day not eating. This type of fasting would reduce calorie intake by over 14 per cent.

A little clarification here. If we decided to fast on Tuesdays, so our last meal was, say, seven pm on Monday evening, and our next would be breakfast on Wednesday morning, at say seven am, then our fast would actually be of 36 hours, which is a long period under normal circumstances.

Therefore, usually, a twenty-four hour fast would consist of the final meal on the Monday, with the next meal being dinner on the Tuesday, which would represent a full twenty-four hours. Various developments from 24-hour fasts have come about, probably the best known being the 5:2 diet. We will look at this in more detail later, but briefly this involves a week split into five days of normal eating, with two days of much reduced calories, for example down to just 500 on these days.

The second form of intermittent fasting is often called time restricted fasting, or TRF. In this, eating is limited to certain hours of the day. A 16:8 mix is often used where a 16 hour fast is combined with an eight-hour period in which meals can be taken. Unfortunately, for the epicures among our readers, that doesn't mean that there can be an eight-hour binge, but in practice it means that a meal is consumed at the beginning and end of the period, usually lunch and dinner.

Of course, this does mean that the commonly held truism that breakfast is the most important meal of the day is challenged, since it is usually breakfast that is lost. However, as we will see later, the theory that we cannot manage without breakfast is one that does not have quite the scientific backing as might be claimed by our elders.

What is actually consumed during the fasting periods is open to discussion. Some say just water (it is very important to remain hydrated). Others will allow beverages such as tea and coffee while, as we see above, some views exist that fasting can be taken to mean drastically reducing our calorie intake, but still eating a little.

Challenging Existing Thinking – Myths And Misconceptions About Intermittent Fasting

Eating Lots of Small Meals Improves Our Metabolism

The idea that consuming lots of small meals will increase our metabolism, making the burning of calories more efficient, is often propounded. It is true that the process of digestion does take up some calories, and the activity in making six meals a day – after all, none of us have lives to live(!) – probably burns a few grapes worth of energy. But what research is proving is that while it is true that the body uses energy during the digestive cycle, called the thermic effect of food (TEF), what matters is the total amount of calories that are consumed.

Eating two meals each of 1200 calories has exactly the same impact as consuming six meals each of four hundred calories.

So, in terms of eating more, smaller, meals to lose weight, the scientific evidence suggests that there will be no obvious benefits.

Eating At Short Intervals Stops Hunger Pangs

This is another theory put forward by the 'many meals' brigade. Because the theory is the basis of many diet programs, studies have been conducted to see whether the claim above is true. The results were mixed, with an even mix between those that suggested that yes, eating less but more often reduces hunger and the craving for calorific snacks. Those that found no impact and those that suggested larger, more spaced out meals reduced snacking.

The best conclusion is to suggest that it is all down to the individual, and if snacking helps, then that can still be fitted into your intermittent fasting plan.

Missing Out on Breakfast Makes Us Fatter

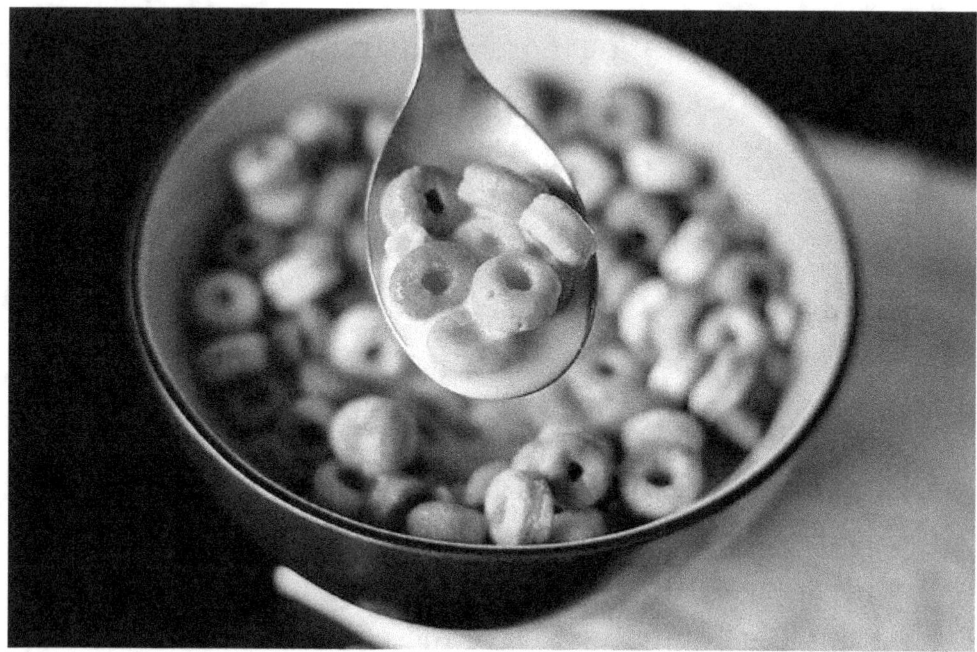

It is certainly true that there appears to be a link; however, studies suggest that this is not to do with missing breakfast, but about all around life style. Those who miss breakfast are, the studies suggest, more likely to indulge in a less healthy lifestyle.

When tests remove this factor, it is discovered that there is no difference at all in body fat increase between those who do eat the early meal of the day, and those who do not.

Just one word of warning here, the above is true with regards to weight, but there have been a number of studies demonstrating that for young people – children and teenagers – breakfast is important for ensuring optimum performance at school.

Fasting Makes the Body Think it is Time to Preserve Calories — thus I won't lose weight if I fast:

There is an often-stated claim that our bodies think fasting is evidence of famine, and therefore stores body fat for later calorie use. Again, as with most myths, there is some truth in this. The condition has a technical name, adaptive thermogenesis.

However, this only applies with full fasting where you go for long protracted periods (Days) without eating. With intermittent fasting, eating is still regular, and there is still a good calorie intake. Your body is amazingly efficient at regulating itself and adapting, so within a few days of intermittent fasting your body will be used to the new regime and no how to expend and store calories and fat accordingly.

Some studies have suggested that intermittent fasting actually increases the body's metabolism, due to an increase in the chemical norepinephrine, which is carried in our blood.

Fasting Intermittently Will Damage Our Health

We will be looking into the considerable advantages of fasting later in the book. However, for now, we can simply say that numerous studies have demonstrated that the claim that there are detrimental health impacts to be experienced from intermittent fasting is without foundation. The science suggests the opposite.

You Cannot Exercise when Fasting

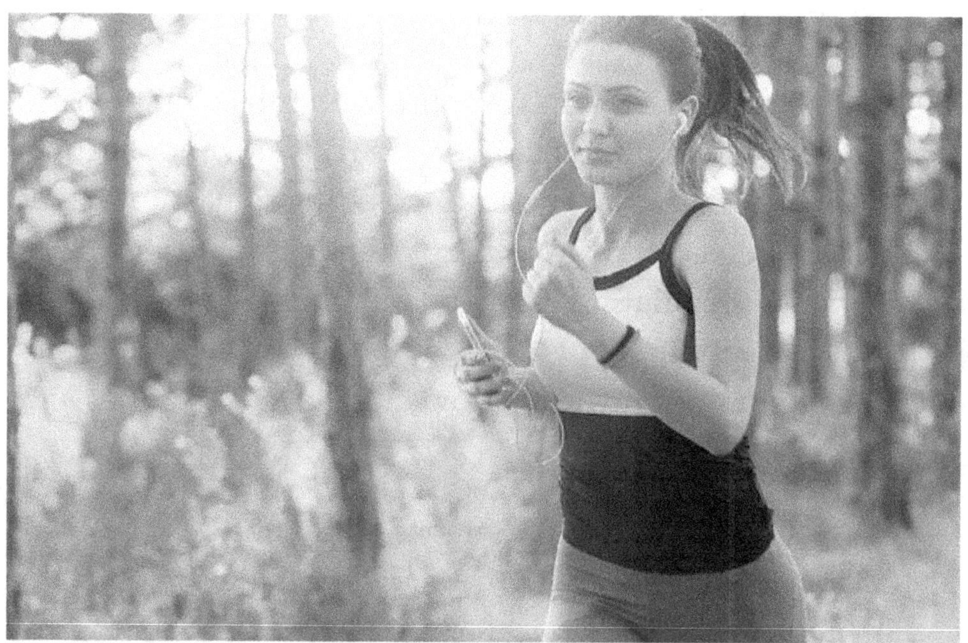

This is yet another old wives' tale with no basis in fact. OK, if we have not eaten for a week, we are going to feel light headed and unwell, but that is a totally different situation to exercising during intermittent fasting. Here, the body is low on glucose, so it burns fat during exercise, suggesting that to undertake a work out before our first post fasting meal is the way of doing it.

In fact, many athletes will only exercise in a state of fast (for example, the morning before eating anything) because this is one of the key steps to reducing your body fat composition and building lean muscle. Want that six pack? Work out in a state of fast because your body will burn carbohydrates and stored fat for fuel to energize your workout instead of those waffles you ate before coming to the gym.

Fasting Leads to Binge Eating

Well, it could. But we have to trust people's common sense. Fasting will lead to an overall drop in calorie consumption, because any extra food we consume during our remaining meals will still be less than the overall intake we used to devour.

Clearly, if we miss breakfast, then have a massive fried lunch, with loads of bread and three desserts, then the fasting will not work. But come on, we can all use our common sense without being nannied.

There are many other myths about intermittent fasting, but the ones above tend to be the most common that are thrown around. We will soon be looking at the science behind this lifestyle choice, and that will put to bed any other unhelpful misconceptions which exist around the subject.

The History Around Intermittent Fasting And The Cultural Importance Of Fasting

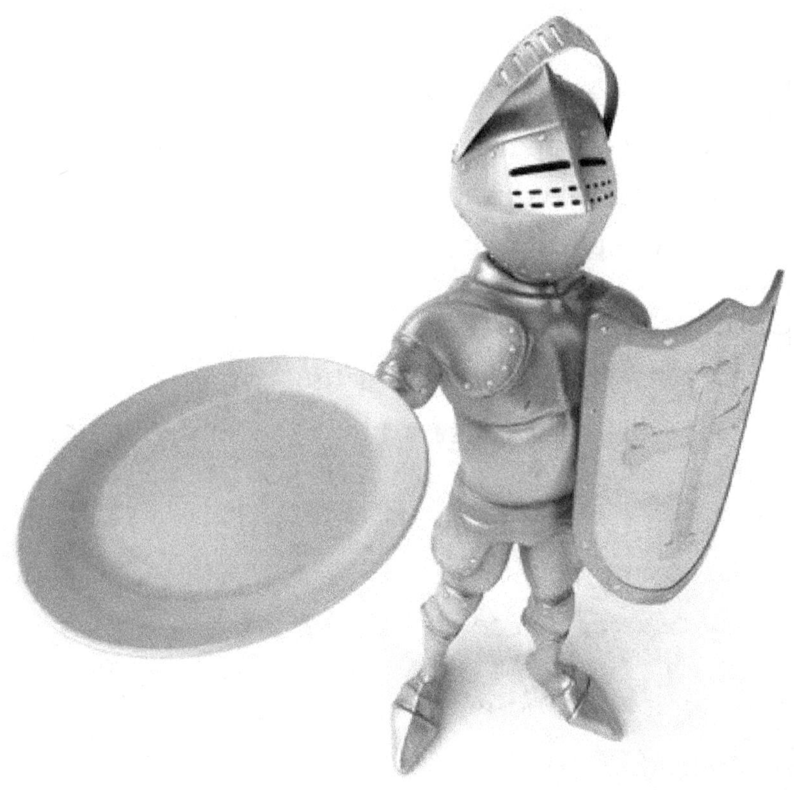

The idea of fasting dates back to primitive cultures in ancient times. Often, before entering a battle, combatants would fast to clear the body and mind of poisons and bad spirits. Coming of age rituals also included fasting, a way to ensure that angry Gods could be expelled from the body, or, in the case of the Native American indigenous population, as a way to mitigate against natural disasters such as famines.

Depending on our beliefs, we probably dismiss the above with a smile, but it cannot be denied that even way back in time our ancestors understood that a fast was a useful tool for the body and the mind.

Of the major world religions, only Zoroastrianism doesn't include fasting among its rituals, in fact it is banned in that particular Eastern belief system. Fasting is associated here with self-control and as a self-penance for sin. In Christianity, people fast leading up to Easter Ramadan is the month of fasting in Islam, Yom Kippur is one of many days of fast celebrated in Judaism.

Surviving a period without sustenance is often viewed as a way of achieving holy insights and purity of body and mind, in a similar way to that celebrated in the primitive cultures mentioned above.

What our forefathers knew was that going without food somehow enhanced the person, made their body feel better, their mind clearer. Today, we can apply science to this, and see that the fast encourages changes into the body to heighten awareness and get rid of fat. But the fact remains that over time fasting has been seen, throughout virtually the entire globe, as a good thing.

But we also know that there is an optimum time for fasting, and that is quite short, rarely more than a day before we should break the fast for at least twenty-four hours. That has led the fast to become a form of protest. IRA who believed that they had been wrongly interred in Northern Ireland would go on hunger strike, occasionally resulting in death. Suffragettes used to fast as a method of protest as they sought suffrage for women in Britain, and other parts of the world. Mahatma Gandhi fasted not once but seventeen times, once for twenty-one days, as he fought for the independence of India from British rule.

Bizarre examples of extreme fasting have also emerged over history. At the turn of the last century an American woman, Linda Burfield – she liked to be known as Doctor Burfield – is thought to have killed no less than forty 'patients' by placing them on strict fasts. It ended with her being convicted of manslaughter. Burfield at least believed in her remedy; she entered a fast of her own in 1938, such an intense one that it led to her own death. During Victorian times, a cult developed of 'Fasting Girls', a group that believed they could live without food.

Doctors tested one, Sarah Jacobs, and discovered upon her death that the claims proved to be groundless. She was just twelve years old.

Let me just take a moment to tell you that the only reason I'm including this is to give you some historical color. Of course you are in no danger of physical harm from intermittent fasting — these people were extremists that did not understand the science behind fasting as we now do.

However, fasting has gone in and out of fashion in the world of health. The Natural Hygiene Movement was developed in the 19th and 20th centuries. Dr Herbert Shelton claimed that his 'Health School' in San Antonio, opened in 1928, cured forty thousand patients. The treatment? Water and fasting.

Indeed, the 1920s marked a high in the use of fasting for medical treatments. The Nature Cure was a UK initiative that stressed the importance of exercise, positive thinking, sunshine and fasting. The UK also boasted fasting clinics at Tyringham Hall and Champneys, which is still open and operating today, although it now runs mainly as an upmarket spa.

Fasting used to be employed to treat a whole range of illness, from heart disease to allergies, from high blood pressure to obesity. The common sense can be seen easily. Reduce fat and many of those diseases reduce or disappear. Since many allergies are caused by food intolerances that increase over time, again fasting would help to address the problem.

Fasting went out of fashion post war, with just small pockets of devotees. However, a resurgence began to hit at the turn of the millennium. The first sign was a website, back in the early days of mass use of the internet. The Warrior Diet was published by Ori Hofmekler in 1999, and just three years later he released the diet as a book. The concept gained more impetus following Brad Pilon's 2006 book, *Eat Stop Eat, with Lean Gains* published by Martin Berkhan a year later.

The growth of the internet into ever wider parts of society meant that Berkhan's book gained a huge following, to the extent that many identify him as being the engine that made fasting popular again. From there, growth has been exponential, perhaps the 5:2 version being most popular.

Fasting is back.

Which People Are Best Suited For Intermittent Fasting, And Who is Not?

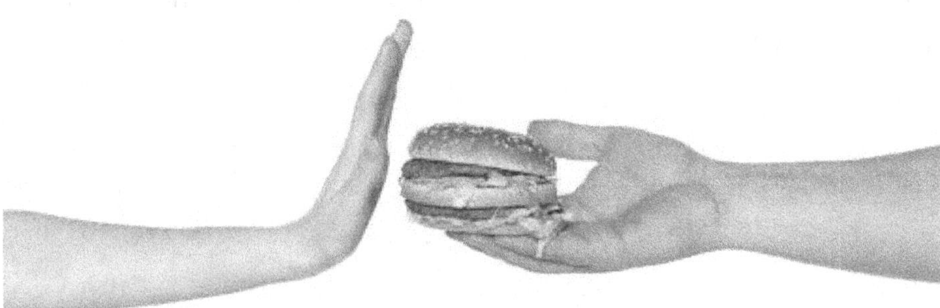

There are not too many people for whom intermittent fasting is unsuitable – we will identify these in a moment. Most people will see weight loss and general health benefits. A degree of will power is needed…but compared to most weight loss routines, not much. After all, if you adopt say the 16:8 diet, then those sixteen hours without food include eight where you are sleeping, so only eight need to be food free. And, during those, you can still drink water, tea, coffee and fresh juices (no sugar added of course).

However, for some people this type of fasting can be really useful for general health matters, even if weight lost is not something in which you are interested. Suffer from inflammation – a sore back for example? Have high blood pressure? Worried about getting Type 2 diabetes? Worried about your heart? Cholesterol too high? Insulin resistance a problem? In all of these examples, intermittent fasting could really help your condition.

Certainly, if you have a pre-existing illness, such as resistance to insulin, then always seek medical advice prior to going onto any form of change to your eating routine. Yet, in all likelihood, you will get the go ahead to start your program.

Research is in its early stages, but there is also a growing body of evidence to suggest that intermittent fasting could be useful in preventing or delaying the onset of dementia illnesses, such as Alzheimer's. There is also some evidence that this type of diet regime could actually make you live longer. After all, healthier people with a good weight live longer than the unhealthy and obese.

However, there are some people for whom intermittent fasting is not appropriate, at least without explicit medical approval. Firstly, fasting is not suitable for young people who are still growing.

Equally, there are some suggestions that it may not be great for the elderly. Of course, such a term is hard to define, but anybody over the age of retirement would be wise to get medical advice before embarking on a program of intermittent fasting.

People with serious pre-existing conditions, such as cancer, heart disease and so forth should get medical advice before starting a program, and those with diabetes should avoid this regime unless their doctors have advised otherwise. Mothers who are breastfeeding, or women who are pregnant, should avoid intermittent fasting – their bodies are adapting for their current life situation, and it is best to trust our bodies in these circumstances.

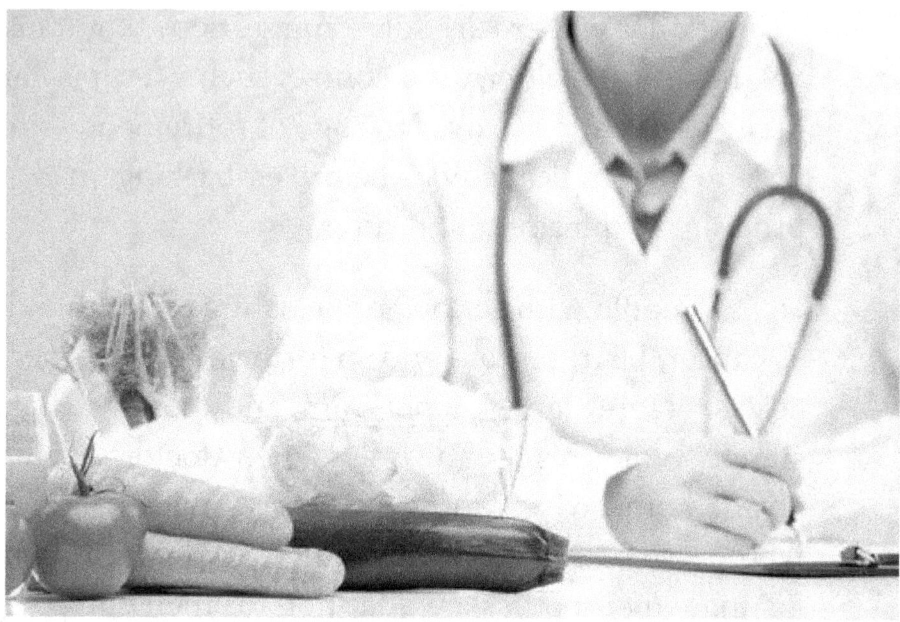

Of course regardless of whether you fit into any of the above categories, if you have any concerns about whether this diet is right for you, you should always talk to your doctor. The above is not an exhaustive list, just some of the more obvious demographics for whom intermittent dieting may not be suitable.

Nevertheless, for the overwhelming majority of people, this diet is a relatively easy method of becoming healthier and losing weight.

Pros And Cons Of Intermittent Fasting

We have covered some of these earlier in the book, so here we will simply outline the main pros and cons so that readers can easily see the body of evidence to help them make a decision as to whether it is something they want to try.

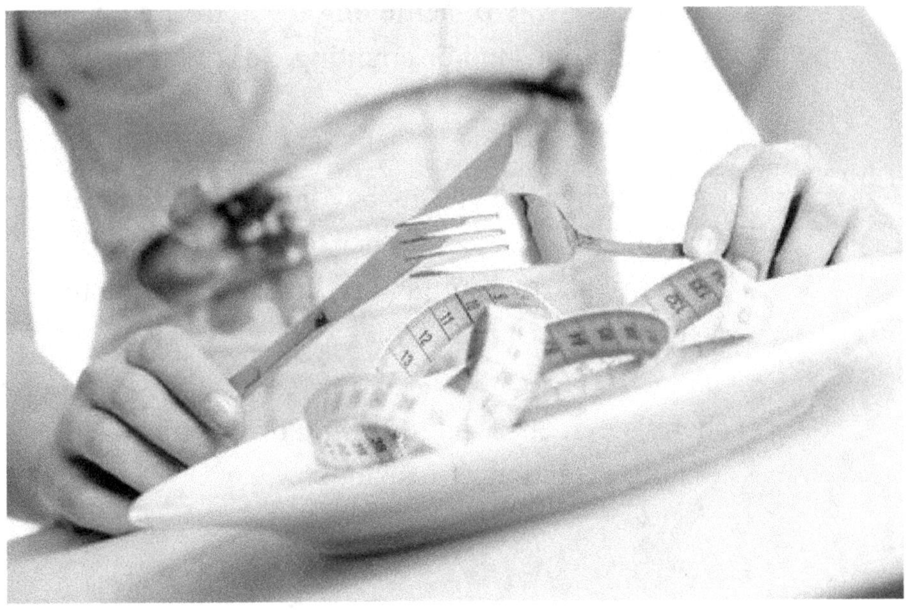

Pros:

- You will almost certainly lose weight.
- Fasting provides a body cleansing service, which can eliminate poisons from the body. (which will

make you feel better, reduce bloating, and reduce your risk of many different types of diseases)

- Because the fasting is reasonable regular, those poisons are less likely to build up.

- It is a cheap way of losing weight and becoming healthier.

- It is an easy way of achieving the above, with no measuring out food or counting calories.

- There are health benefits beyond weight loss. Evidence suggests a number of conditions will be eased by intermittent fasting, and it can delay the onset of others.

- There is evidence that this kind of fasting can actually extend our lifespan.

- There are many types of intermittent fasting, which means that we can select one that best fits our lifestyle and personality.

- You can eat what you want to eat, which makes it easier to keep up.

- Evidence suggests that our bodies adapt very quickly to this kind of fasting, which makes it easier to keep up. We all know the problem of other kinds of diet, where we can crave foods we are not allowed to eat.

- Our overall calorie intake will go down.

- Some evidence suggests that it can increase concentration and mental focus, making our work better.

- Because we feel healthy, our moods are more consistent and better, improving personal relationships.

- The diet is compatible with exercise programs.

- Fasting can be a short-term fix, or a long-term lifestyle choice. Both methods will provide some benefit.

- Fasting has, for many years, formed a part of the culture of various societies.

Cons

- Some will power is needed to keep up the regime, particularly in the early stages.
- Intermittent fasting is not suitable for some groups of people. See above for details or speak with your doctor prior to undertaking the regime.
- Although it is growing, the body of scientific research into this type of diet is still limited.
- Some people can suffer energy dips during fasting days, which can lead to dizziness, fuzziness of thought and mood swings, at least in the early stages of a program.
- Hormone change can occur, especially in women, if too much fasting is undertaken.
- Those with eating disorders can find their conditions worsen if they fast.
- There are some reports that suggest a higher incidence of injuries during exercise can occur.

As is clearly evident, the strengths and benefits of intermittent fasting far outweigh possible problems. Most of the negatives will apply to only a small number of users of the diet and provided medical advice is sought where needed, people will see very positive results from entering into a program.

Chapter Summary

In this chapter we have looked at the following areas.

- We have defined exactly what intermittent fasting is and seen that it can take many forms.

- We have debunked some of the common myths and misconceptions about the idea, seeing that for the majority of people, there are no risks and considerable potential benefits.

- We have seen the cultural history of fasting and come to understand that it forms a part of almost every culture and religion across the globe.

- From the turn of the millennium, we have seen how it has come back in fashion, really for the first time since the 1920's, but with more research behind it.

- For the majority of people, as we have seen, this diet regime offers a safe and practical way to lose weight and become healthier. However, for some age groups and for those suffering from certain health related conditions, intermittent fasting may not be suitable.

- We have seen that there are considerable benefits beyond just weight loss, although there are a smaller number of negatives that may apply to a small number of people.

In the next chapter we will learn about the science underpinning the concept of intermittent fasting.

Chapter Two: The Growing Body Of Scientific Evidence

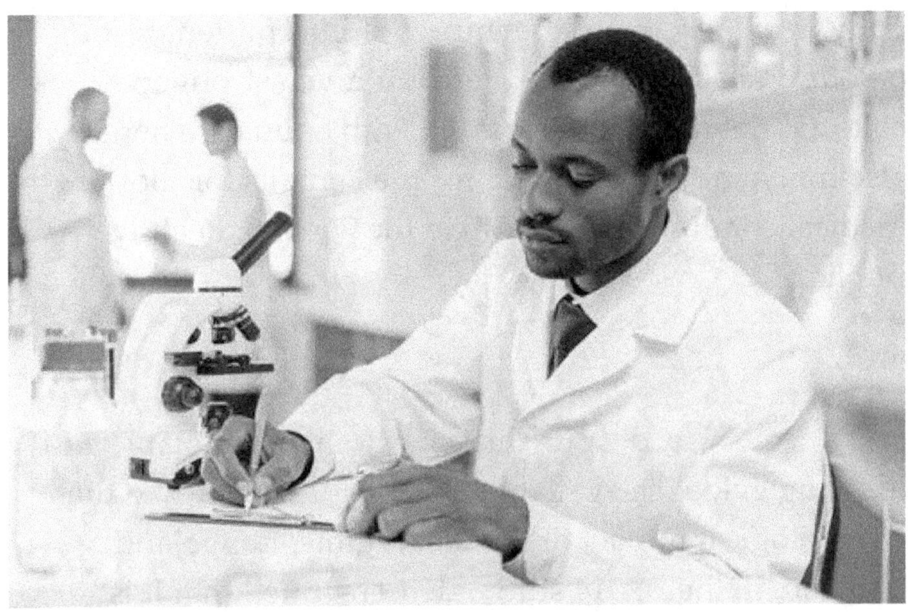

In this chapter we will examine the research undertaken in the scientific community about intermittent fasting. Then, we will see the biological and chemical changes that result in the body when a regime is begun. Finally, we will look at its impact on metabolism.

Scientific Research And Evidence

As we have stated earlier, there is still only a small body of evidence into the impact of intermittent fasting on our bodies. However, there is a much stronger collection of data from research with animals. There is also much greater evidence for the benefits for those with medical conditions, rather than the general, healthy public.

However, despite this caveat, there is reliable and growing evidence available. Some of this relates to the psychological impact of the diet regime. Longo and Mattson, in their 2014 study, demonstrated that it is relatively easy to get used to the new way of eating. However, the first three to six weeks can be tough. Get through that, and the body becomes used to the method, and hunger pangs and cravings disappear. So, this suggests that the first few weeks are crucial.

Research by Ganley as far back as 1989, before the resurgence in the popularity of this kind of fasting, supported the views of Longo and Mattson, but in a different way. Ganley discovered that people mostly change their *views* towards hunger, while it still exists. The findings were that people undertaking this kind of diet recognized hunger but saw it in a positive light. They saw it as a sign of pride and success, indicating that their diet was working. Normally, feelings of hunger can trigger panic, or desire.

Since we know that such hunger exists for only a short time, the impact found by Ganley means that most people get through it well, making the diet much easier to adhere to than many others.

However, more recent research has challenged Ganley's findings, suggesting that these early days can be tougher than just experiencing hunger. Loss of libido, mood swings and further negative effects were identified by, among others, Johnstone in 2007. However, all of these studies concluded that any negatives are short lived.

The conclusion that we can draw from the research into the psychological effects of this kind of lifestyle choice is that the first few weeks are likely to be tough, but not for everybody. Some negatives could well be experienced in these early days, but they will be short lived, and then the body (and so the mind) will adapt and cope with ease.

The medical benefits of intermittent fasting can be traced back in experiments of over eighty years ago. In the 1930's, McCay published a paper on the impact of occasional fasting in the lifespan of rats. It concluded that the process lengthened the rodents' lives. Since then, numerous studies have demonstrated the same, although most of these have been limited to smaller mammals or other animal types.

A study in 2009 by Mattson demonstrated an interesting impact in monkeys. It found that overall there was not definite increase in life span, but where a monkey did live beyond average, it did so by a considerable amount. It also found that the group who underwent the intermittent fasting regime were healthier, even when their life was not extended.

Some tests have examined the lifestyle of certain groups of people. On Okinawa Island, a part of Japan, older citizens follow an ancient mantra – 'hara hachi bu' which translates as 'eat until four fifths full. While there could be other factors, such as the high fish content of their diet, the people of Okinawa Island have the highest percentage of people living beyond 100 out of anywhere in the world.

Other tests involving humans have found similar results to the Mattson test with primates. Weight reduction, improved insulin absorption, lower blood pressure and cholesterol and so forth. However, those tests have tended to be carried out on people who are already considered obese.

The aforementioned Mattson, who is a professor of neuroscience, has conducted specific research into the impact of fasting on the health of the brain. He discovered that limiting calorie intake on at least two days per week will improve connections in the hippocampus part of the brain.

It also helps the brain to defend against the proteins that build up to cause diseases such as Parkinson's and Alzheimer's. For Mattson, there is a common sense, historical point to the benefits to the brain that are created by fasting. He believes that historically, times of famine (which necessitated fasting) required the brain to be at its clearest and most efficient, in order to maximize the opportunities to find food.

Our brains have evolved to function best during times when food is limited. However, Mattson advises that the best way to self-induce fasting, rather than have it thrust upon us, is to start slowly. Rather like when we take up exercise after a long period of not doing much physically, we need to build up to our full fasting program, rather than diving straight into it.

The conclusion of the evidence on the physical impacts of intermittent fasting on the body seems to be that weight will be lost, health will be improved, and some medical conditions will be delayed. There may be an overall increase in life expectancy as a result of the improved health of participants, but there will be definitely be an improved quality of life irrespective of whether it is extended or not.

Biological And Chemical Changes In The Body During Fasting

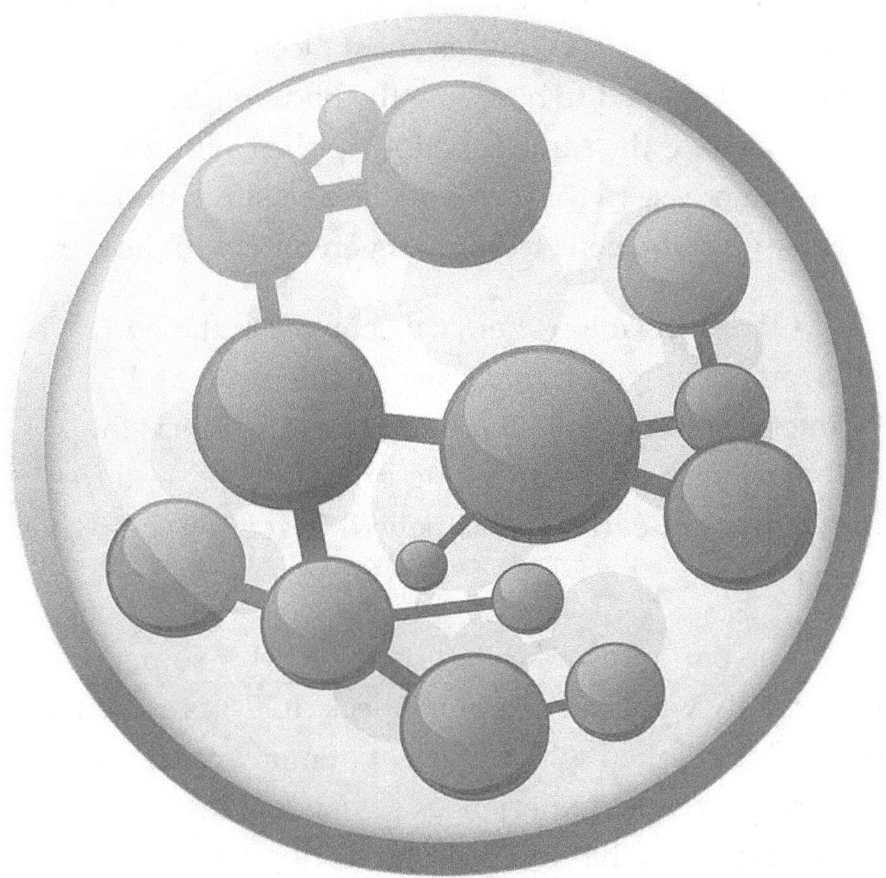

One of the first biological changes to occur is that blood pressure drops, by about ten percent. This has obvious positive health impacts, although research suggests at the moment that the pressure returns to its previous state when the fasting stops.

Another impact is more mysterious. A characteristic of blood, called – vaguely – an 'embryonic like substance' – increases. Scientists are still unsure exactly what function this part of our blood performs. There is more evidence of this substance in animals, where it is believed to be a way the body repairs itself from disease. If the same function applies in humans, then the increase in this can only be a positive thing. It will enable blood cells to allow regeneration in the body.

One of the main chemical changes in the body we find from fasting is an increase in a chemical inhibitor, the interestingly named IGFBP-1. Broadly, this is the inhibitor which keeps the aging process stable and free from disease. Clearly, such a benefit is going to help us as we get older.

The part of us inhibited by IGFBP-1 is something we certainly want to be kept in check. IGF-1 is a chemical in our blood linked with the onset of many cancers, and other negatives we experience as we get older. Therefore, the conclusion is that intermittent fasting will protect us from many diseases.

Another change in the body is a reduction in the 'addiction' chemicals the brain produces. It seems as though dopamine, the chemical which gives a feeling of satisfaction, is repressed to some extent, which could have a benefit for addictions, such as certain foods, and even alcohol and nicotine.

As with other areas in this field, research is currently limited, and therefore conclusions are far from certain. However, glutamate and GABA, the chemicals which transfer messages to the brain, may be affected, reducing the crave impact of endorphins. In contrast, other scientists, such as consultant psychiatrist Dr Jonathon Chick, are less sure, feeling that personality probably plays a bigger part in addiction.

It must be remembered that the research is still in its early stages with regards to the internal workings of the body, and therefore the conclusions regarding the impact of intermittent fasting are not certain, but the evidence is growing that it really helps us to stay healthy and free from many of the worst diseases to which mankind is exposed – not only in the present but as we get older as well.

The Metabolic Changes Caused By Intermittent Fasting

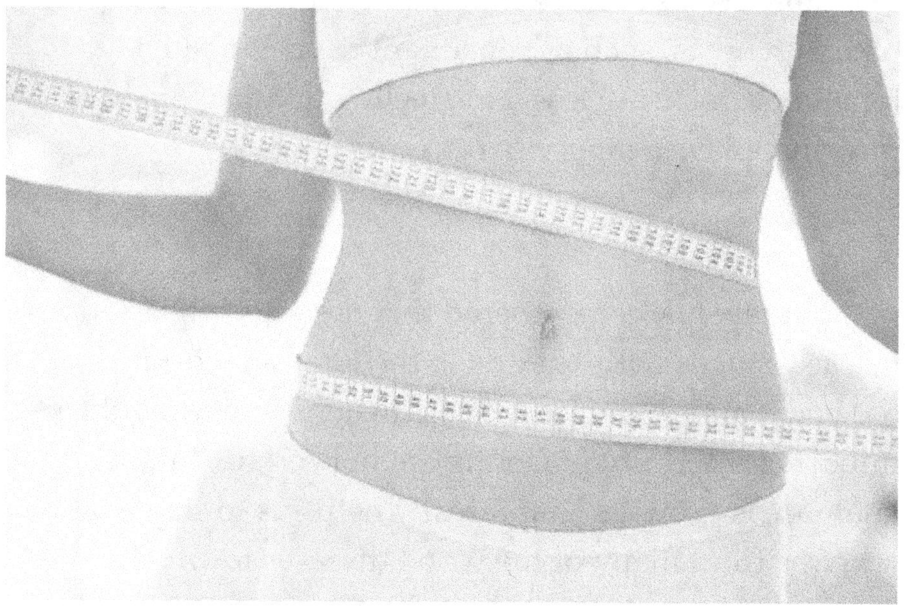

It does seem as though the changes to the metabolism during intermittent fasting are good. Some of the negatives of traditional diets are lost, such as the body losing lean body mass. With this type of fasting, the body attacks stored fat, which it burns to sustain energy levels.

A key part of sustaining and improving your metabolism is the 'intermittent' part of the term. If we fast for too long, then (as we saw earlier) the body can enter starvation mode, where the metabolism slows, and fat is actually stored rather than burned. But as long as we are eating regularly – a 5:2 or 16:8 approach both work perfectly, then the metabolism will increase.

Studies into the effect of Ramadan, the Muslim holy fasting month, on metabolism have indicated that if you fast for sixteen hours, or more, then your metabolism increases. However, that lasts for seventy hours, after which it returns to normal, then quickly slows.

All in all, then, we can see that there is strong evidence for the health benefits of intermittent fasting, biologically, chemically and metabolically.

Chapter Summary

We have seen in this chapter that:

- Scientific research is limited, but growing, regarding humans; but much exists for animals, which seems likely to be transferrable to humans.
- The body soon gets used to fasting, although in the early stages it may be tough.
- There is strong evidence regarding the health benefits of fasting.
- Fasting for up to 72 hours is good for the metabolism, however sixteen and twenty-four hours can achieve this effect without huge discomfort.

In the next chapter you will learn in detail about the benefits we have already identified as coming from intermittent fasting.

Chapter Three: A Detailed Look At the Benefits Offered Through Intermittent Fasting

In this chapter we will revisit some of the biggest benefits we can get from intermittent fasting and look at them in much greater detail.

Weight Loss

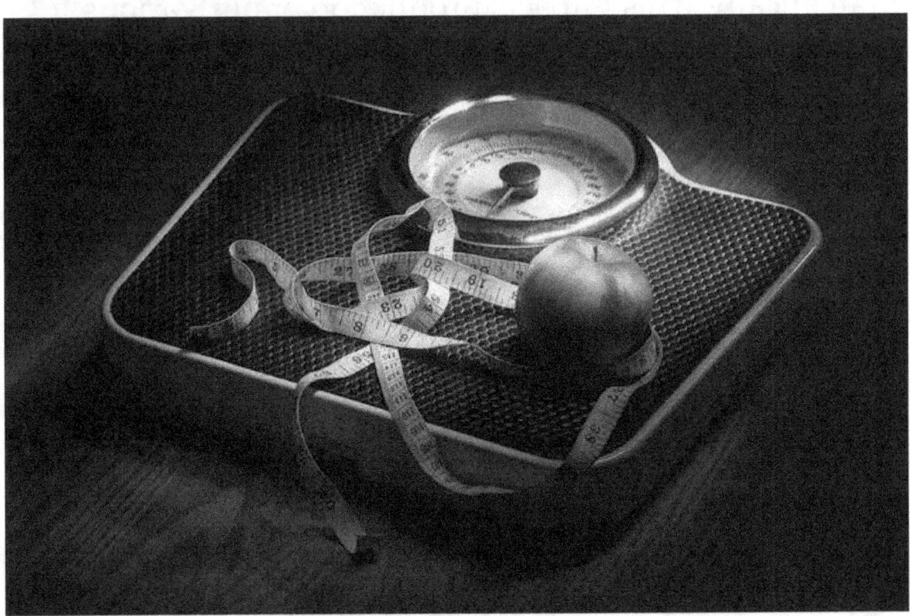

Many people have seen their weight drop significantly after following an intermittent fasting diet for a short while. Perhaps more importantly, they have seen that weight stay off. This is because fasting alters the way the body works with food. Under normal circumstances, fat is stored for 'emergency use'.

The body gets its energy from converting food into glucose-based substances. If that glucose is your body's current bank account, then fat is its long-term savings policy, which needs a number of criteria satisfied before it can access those reserves. Fasting is the key that meets those conditions.

When we fast, our insulin levels decrease dramatically. This impacts production of our various glucose substances and therefore the body begins to employ its stored body fats for its energy. When we use those fats, our waistline reduces in size and our weight begins to drop.

Another reason we lose weight when we fast is due to our human growth hormone rising. It can increase as much as five times its normal level. The hormone helps us gain muscle and lose fat. HGH or human growth hormone helps the body to burn fat – it peaks during puberty then decreases from then on. It is present in adults, although in much lower amounts which decrease with age. If we can increase those levels of HGH – the like we do through intermittent fasting– we burn more fat and lose weight.

Meanwhile, our brain is trying to figure out what's going on. There it is, expecting a bowl of cereal, a couple of eggs and a sausage and instead it receives…a glass of water. The result is that the brain moves from out of its inert state of DefCon 5 up to level four and employs its first line of defense against starvation. It instructs our nervous system to release norepinephrine to the fat cells. This makes the fat cells break down our body fat to release it. The body then burns this for its energy.

Another factor in intermittent fasting leading to weight loss is that, overall, we tend to eat fewer calories. Through the processes explained above, when our calorie intake falls, our bodies move to our stored fat to get its energy.

If we imagine that we are using a 5:2 regime, we can see how this works.

An average man will need around 17,500 calories per week; a woman around 14,000. This works out to be 2500 per day for a man, with 2000 for a woman. We can assume that this is an average of say 700 calories for breakfast and lunch, with perhaps 900 calories for the main meal of the day. This leaves around two hundred for snacks and incidentals. A woman will consume slightly less at each meal. That is actually quite a lot of food.

Let us take the example of a man to illustrate the point of how intermittent fasting reduces our overall calorie intake. In the 5:2 diet, for two days out of seven, calorie intake is limited to 500 per day. That leaves 16,500 for the remaining five days, or 3300 per day. In other words, eight hundred calories on top of our normal recommended consumption per day. We will not be increasing our normal meals by between a third and a half, even though they might be slightly bigger, especially in the day after the fast. On top of this, remember that we saw earlier that the body quickly gets used to the new regime, and there are not hunger pangs.

Overall, although we may not save the full 4000 calories by fasting, we will probably save 3000 of them, more than a day's calorie intake.

Health Benefits

The second major reason for embarking on a program of intermittent fasting is for the health benefits that are gained.

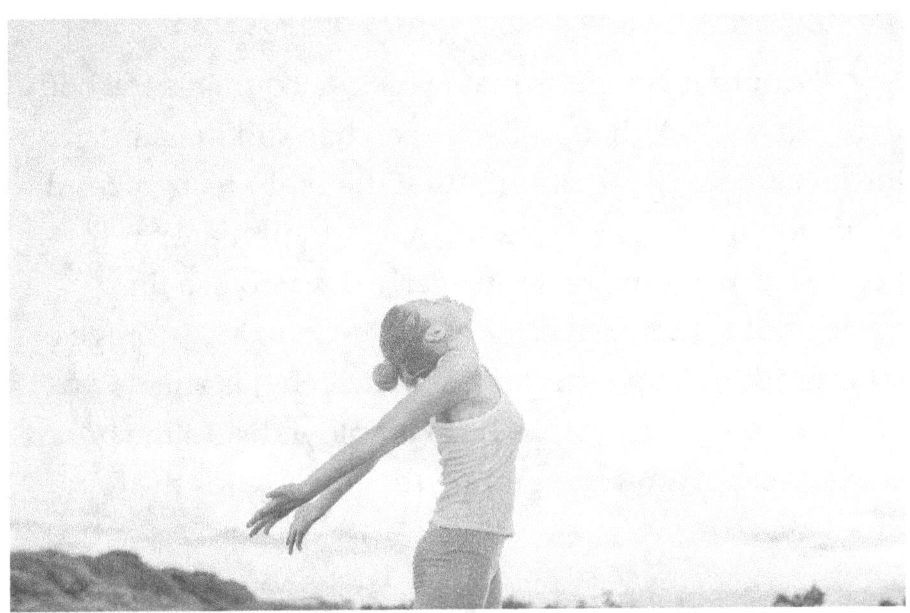

Some of this can be understood because they are common sense. If fasting allows us to burn more body fat, then our body has less fat to clog up arteries and cause heart problems.

If we are obese, then we are more susceptible to a range of conditions from diabetes to cancer. Through fasting, we eliminate obesity, and greatly reduce our risk of those health conditions (diabetes, cancer etc). Scientifically speaking, fasting actually reduces the production of the harmful type of cholesterol, LDL. Inflammation is also prevented, which helps our internal organs remain healthier. This includes the heart, lungs, kidneys, liver and so on.

Another benefit is that fasting encourages the body to repair cells. Although the research is still in its infancy, the belief among scientists is that the brain recognizes the reduction in caloric intake and starts to prepare for the possibility of a famine. In the early days, to use the analogy of earlier in the chapter, DefCon One (storage of fat caused by long term calorie deficiency) is still a way off, but DefCon Three has been employed, and the brain starts to clean out cells, getting them ready for the tough times ahead.

This directs some its energy to the repairing cells, which in turn leads to an overall improvement in health.

Another related change is that some of the body's genes change (particularly the ones related to longevity and disease resistance). Our bodies have changed from their normal laid-back state to fighting machines ready for the perceived battles ahead. Of course, as we know, the brain is a bit mistaken, because the only thing we'll be battling is calories– we will neither enter famine nor will we suffer severe impacts from cravings or hunger…our brains aren't as smart as they think they are, but that's just our little secret.

As we saw earlier, some research suggests that fasting can delay or prevent the onset of some brain conditions such as Alzheimer's and Parkinson's disease. Research has demonstrated that fasting can increase the life span of animals by as much as fifty per cent. It has also discovered that intermittent fasting delivers the same results in animals as the results achieved from continuous fasting, where just a minimum of necessary calories are consumed. This means you can achieve the same results much more painlessly, and without posing any risk to your health (unlike continuous fasting). Scientists think that this results because of the following: It seems as though dropping calories causes the brain to trigger protective actions in itself. DefCon Four!

Going back to Professor Mattson, who as head of neuroscience at the US National Institute on Aging, he explains that fasting produces a similar reaction in the brain to exercise (imagine, then, what can be gained from doing both!) At the moment, we are still learning what causes brain diseases such as Alzheimer's, but a factor definitely seems to be brain shrinkage which grows with age. Cells die off, which is a normal life process. It is just that, when we are younger, they are replaced by new ones. That regeneration decreases with age.

However, as Professor Mattson explains, when we are obese, the hormones ghrelin and leptin are less effective. Since part of their job is to grow new brain cells, this is a bit of a problem. The weight loss and fat loss benefit of intermittent fasting means that these hormones remain more active, creating more brain cells to reduce the ones lost through natural aging.

Yet Another major health benefit to be gained from fasting is the diabetes prevention. This condition is one of the major problems of the western world. Our high sugar diets, and astronomical levels of obesity have led to a surge in type two diabetes. This condition can lead to some conditions we really do not want to experience. Diabetes accounts for the biggest group of people to lose their sight during adulthood. It can lead to a hardening of the arteries, which can cause heart disease. Such a condition is made worse by high cholesterol and high blood pressure, conditions also associated with obesity.

Diabetes can lead to poor circulation, in the worst cases leading to the need for amputation, usually of the leg or legs. It means the body's natural defense against infection is reduced, and common conditions such as the flu can develop complications, sometimes resulting in death.

Overall, those with diabetes have a lower life expectancy and experience a lower quality of life while they are living.

Diabetes works by reducing the body's sensitivity to insulin. Insulin controls the way the body converts sugars into energy. When our bodies are not responding properly, sugars are not absorbed into energy effectively and instead enter the blood stream where they harden, causing the problems mentioned above.

Fasting increases our sensitivity to insulin and that means that we convert our sugars successfully helping to prevent the onset of Type 2 diabetes.

However, the benefits may be even greater than this. Some research is beginning to suggest that fasting can actually eliminate the disease. Again, research is sketchy at the moment. But, a recent trial of a small number of diabetic patients in the UK's University of Newcastle demonstrated that an eight week fast of 800 calories per day actually reversed the condition in a number of participants.

That sort of caloric intake over such a period would be a challenge, but the benefits to those suffering from diabetes are astonishing to report. Those with diabetes throughout the world wait eagerly for the results of further research.

Another of the many ways in which fasting helps with health is especially applicable to older people. The release of higher levels of HGH mean that bone density is sustained. In many older people, bones become fragile and brittle. The sort of fall a child would bounce up from can lead to fractures and breaks of hips, shoulders, ankles and knees from which, sadly, some elderly people never recover. Thus, the benefits of increased bone density that can be obtained from intermittent fasting could be most transformative.

Increase In Muscle Density

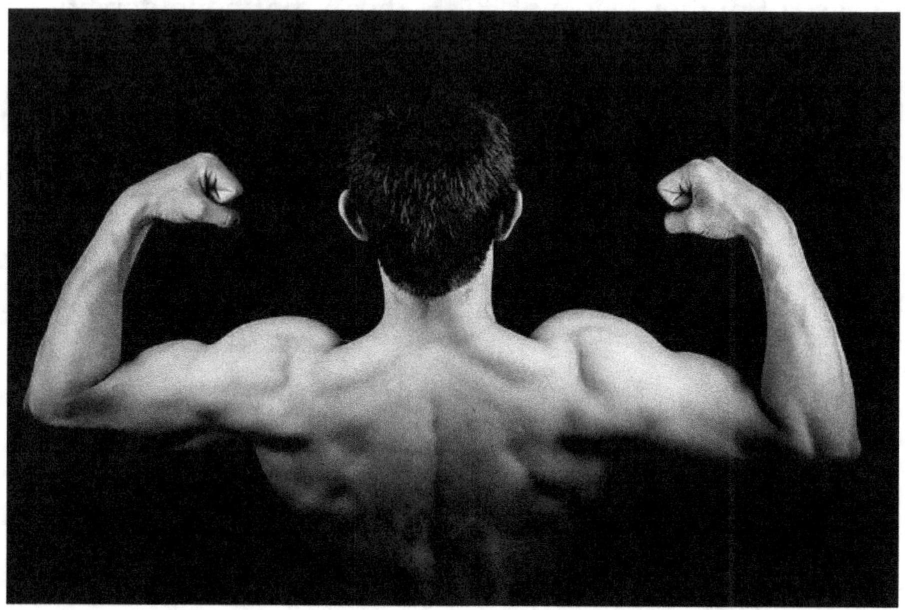

The increased levels of HGH created by intermittent fasting have another benefit, one which was actually behind the resurgence in the regime back in the early 2000s.

It has been widely observed that fasting increases the amount of lean body mass – muscles increase in those who fast intermittently. The early innovators of the resurgence, such as the authors Brad Pilon and Martin Berkhan, were mostly interested in muscle mass as they were keen proponents of body building.

We can see that fasting not only helps us to reduce weight, but also to build and strengthen muscles.

Psychological Benefits

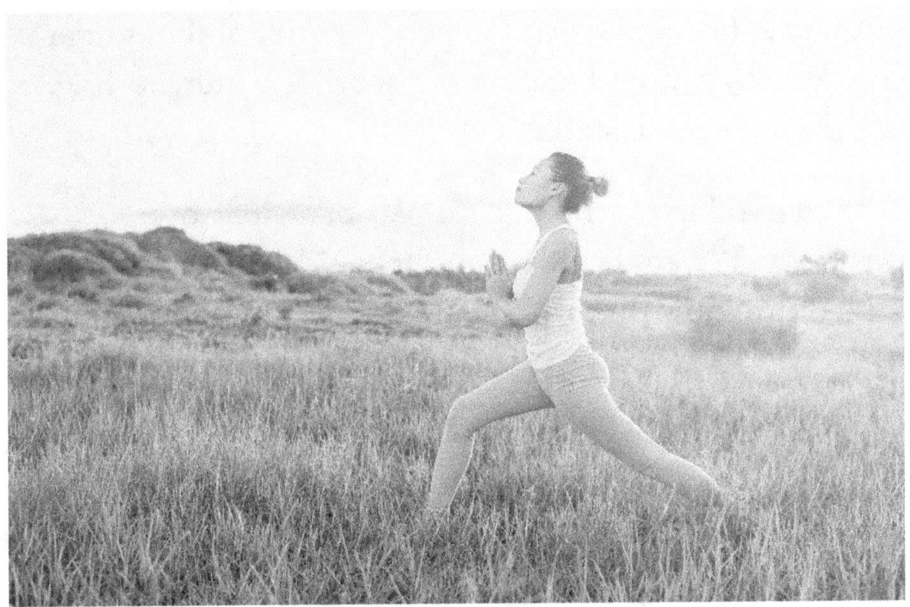

There are numerous psychological benefits we can gain from intermittent fasting. Paramount among them is the fact that we feel and look better. Very few people like being overweight, and most people like the additional energy and buzz of having a healthy body.

On top of this is the sense that we are doing ourselves good. Pride might be one of the deadly sins, but there is no reason why we shouldn't, in a quiet, private moment, take joy in the way we are helping ourselves to be healthy.

Craving hormones are reduced and 'happy' hormones – endorphins – are more apparent in a healthy body. We know that fasting helps to improve clarity of thought and concentration, and therefore our work is better, adding to our feeling of satisfaction.

Feeling good in our minds is a part of a circle of positivity. We are positive, and that aids us in sticking with our regime. In turn, that makes us feel better still.

Easy To Stick With

While researching this book, I decided (on a whim) to google the term 'diets'. Fourteen and a half million articles later, I did feel quite informed about the subject, if a little tired…and hungry. Actually, I have a confession to make, I didn't actually read them all. I know, I know, that's a shocking revelation, but none of us are perfect (despite claims to the contrary from some.)

We are not suggesting that there are fourteen and a half million different diets out there (a surprisingly round number, I am sure you will agree. I remember Google as being more precise in the past) but there are certainly quite a few. It's so overwhelming. And some of these diets are SO hard to implement into your life. It makes my head hurt just reading about them.

In reality, unless we have a medical condition that stops us, it is pretty easy to lose weight. The answer is to burn more calories than you take in. On that basis, this book could have been just two sentences long. But there is a problem. And that is…sadly…us. Atkins diet, Keto diet, Paleo diet, hips and thighs diet…with minor variations, they all do the same thing – reduce our calorie intake. If we add exercise to the formula for calorie intake (more out than in) we develop muscle strength and use even more calories. Our metabolism speeds up, so we digest food before we can turn it into fat.

This is exactly the same for intermittent fasting. As I have stressed to point out, what we are basically doing is reducing our calorie intake, so we then lose weight. We then get all the other benefits, some (but not all) come simply with weight loss.

So, where do we go wrong? The answer is easy, we stick to the diet…for a week or two. Then we return to our old habits. Or, we have a great week and decide to celebrate at the weekend. Half an hour later, we are regretting the triple cheeseburger, supersize fries, extra-large chocolate milk shake etc. In fact, such is our sadness that the only way to cheer us up is to consume a carton of ice cream, with extra fudge and whipped cream.

And that is where intermittent fasting scores so highly. As we have seen with the research carried out on the body adapting to fasting, we quickly fall into line with the regime. But this begs the question as to why we can do this with intermittent fasting, but not other diets. The answer is most probably a combination of several things.

First, it is really easy to implement. We do not need to seek out strange ingredients for our food, we do not need to have miniscule portions that would probably leave most people feeling worse – unsatisfied emotionally as well as physically. We do not have to weigh ingredients or cut out carbohydrates from our food.

If we want six pieces of toast for breakfast, we can have them. Whereas, with some other diets…well, as nice as mashed cauliflower might be, it can wear thin.

With intermittent fasting, when you really want that nice mound of fluffy mashed potatoes, topped with butter to go with your chicken and gravy, then no problem. Chopping up carrots and dipping into a teaspoon of low fat hummus might make us feel virtuous, but not necessarily full. And virtue is a sensation best felt in small doses.

Intermittent fasting just means missing the occasional meal, not building your whole life around the needs of a diet. And that is why people find it easy to stick with. If you are planning to start, just remember to start slowly, and get through the first two or three weeks, and the diet will become a part of your life, not your life becoming a part of the diet.

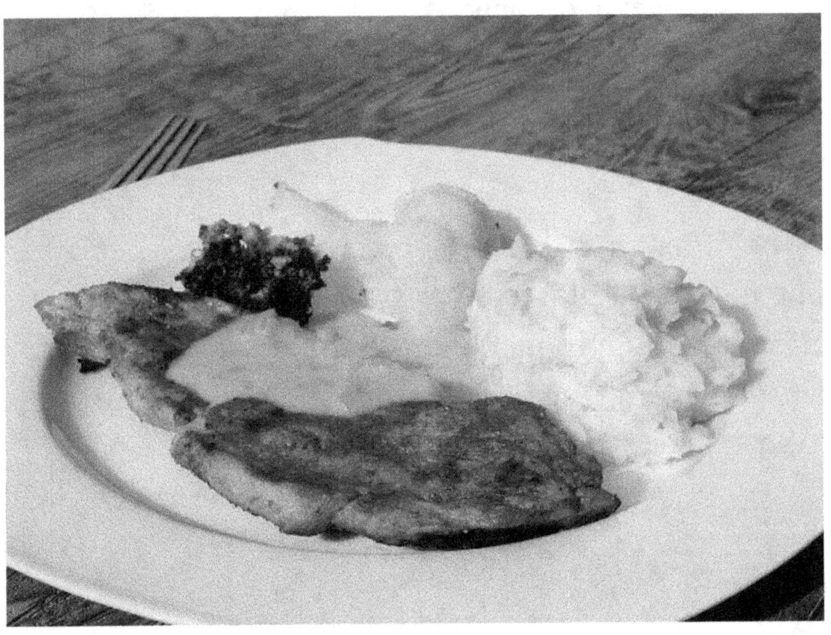

Chapter Summary

In this chapter we have looked in some details at a selection of the many benefits of intermittent fasting.

- The health benefits are manifold.
- There are several mental health and well-being advantages.
- Because our lean body mass increases, we become stronger and leaner.
- The lifestyle is easy to adapt to and keep up.

One of the other strengths on which we did not spend any time in this chapter is the incredible flexibility of intermittent fasting. In fact, we will devote a whole chapter to this, offering detail into many of the various forms it can take.

Chapter Four: Types of Intermittent Fasting

We will look at a number of the ways in which we can use intermittent fasting to improve our health and well-being. Specifically, we will consider the 5:2 method, Leangains, sometimes called the 16:8 version; the alternate day approach, with its UpDayDownDay variation, the Eat-Stop-Eat method, the Warrior Diet, the Fat Loss Forever approach and spontaneous meal skipping.

The Five:Two Method

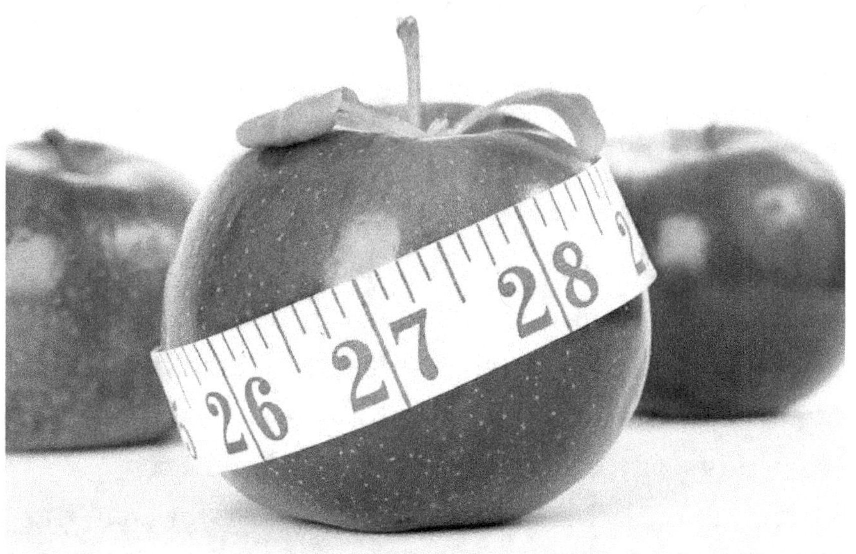

The principle behind this approach is that we eat normally for five days of the week and choose two (non-consecutive) days to eat a much-reduced calorie intake. One of the great advantages of this method is the flexibility it offers.

We can pick which two days we like to fast. For example, many people might want to keep their weekends normal, and might sense that their energy levels begin to drop after a week at work. So fasting days of Monday and Wednesday could work very well for them.

The best idea on the fasting days is to aim for two very light meals, perhaps two meals of 300 calories for men, 250 for women. To give an idea, a breakfast of 300 calories looks a bit like a whole wheat English muffin, topped with low fat butter, a small hard-boiled egg, a handful of fruits and a small glass of fruit juice, plus as much water as you want.

A baked potato with sour cream and a water melon side would make a decent dinner at this number of calories, as would a small chicken breast, grilled and served with some green beans and a small side salad.

Lunch could be a bowl of soup with some saltine crackers, or a roasted vegetable salad with a sweet potato, some greens, pepper and eggplant and a light honey dressing. While these are not huge meals, unsurprisingly at their calorie limits, they are still things we might eat anyway for a meal.

On the remaining five   days of the week we eat normally, three well balanced meals and a snack. In fact, the portions could be a little bigger if we want, especially for meals following a fasting day. As long as the overall weekly calorie intake is lower than normal, the fast will have the effects we seek.

At the time of writing, there have been no specific studies into the 5:2 diet, but we do know that this is a form of intermittent dieting, and that in itself has some research and lots of anecdotal evidence into its benefits.

The 5:2 diet is a great introduction to intermittent fasting. It is a lot less severe than, say the alternate day method, and is therefore quite easy to get into.

Leangains, Or The 16:8 Approach

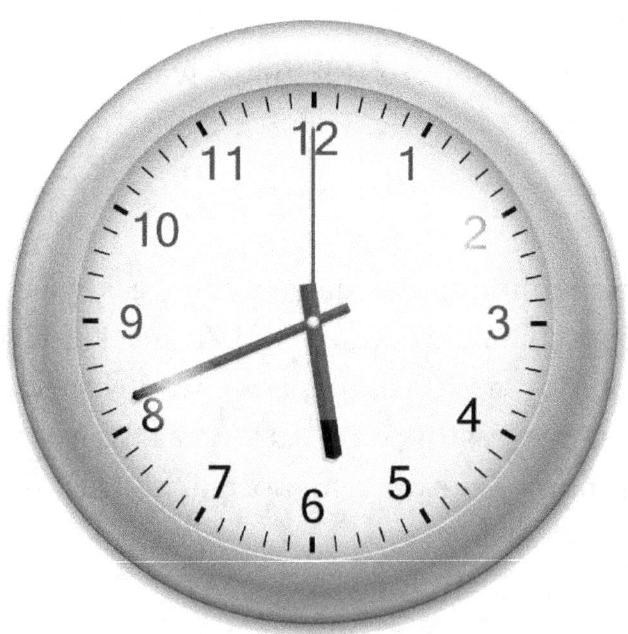

If the 5:2 approach to intermittent fasting is an easy way to get involved in the program, then the 16:8 version is at least as straightforward. Two nice sized meals are eaten every day, and the body very quickly gets used to the fasting part of the day, particularly as it usually includes eight hours of sleep. In fact, some proponents argue that the eating time can be extended from eight to ten hours. On this basis, there are only six hours of waking time per day when you cannot eat.

Many experts in the field believe that it is after around sixteen hours that most people's bodies enter the 'fasting state'. There does seem, though, to be a slight difference between the genders, with women needing around 14-15 hours to reach their optimum fasting state, men slightly longer.

Leangains was made popular by the fitness expert, Martin Berkhan, in the mid '90's. It really is a no-pain way to improve health and lose weight. First, the fasting state is not especially onerous. Most people will follow the program below, but so long as the fasting period is continuous, it can be adapted to best fit an individual's lifestyle.

Let us start with the evening meal. For most people, this is going to be between 7.00 and 8.00pm. We can say for the purposes of this example that we finish eating at 8.00pm. We then relax and go to bed at, say 11.00pm. A good night's sleep and we are up at 7.00am. Our body will soon get used to not having breakfast, and as we saw earlier, the old adage that breakfast is the most important meal of the day does not have much in the way of science to back it up.

In fact, lots of us already skip this meal, although often not for dietary reasons but because we cannot get ourselves together in the morning. We are the people who then overdo it with other meals – if we could get those under control, our bodies would really experience the benefits. And, we can all reassure ourselves that lunch is not far away.

But there is a plus: with the 16:8 diet: it is fine to have a tea or coffee (even with a splash of milk) in that intervening period. A good cup of Americano (try it black, if you don't already have it that way. The taste is soon acquired, and you will wonder why you ever added milk.), or a green tea will see any lingering pangs of hunger firmly in the background as we make our way through morning, head clear and able to work at pace.

A good lunch, we can have a bigger one than normal if we need it, will keep us going through to dinner in the evening. But, if your body tells you so, as we are not in our fasting period, then a late afternoon snack can keep us buzzing until the main meal of the day.

We have said it often, but it bears repeating. The meals in our non-fasting period can be a little bigger than normal, especially as our body is acclimating to its new regime, but they do still need to be healthy and in moderation. Not small, but remember our aim is to reduce our overall calorie intake. The odd take-away is fine, but a week of curries, Chinese take-away, take out pizzas and a giant spread of Mexican food will be as harmful to us during our intermittent fasting as it would be to anybody not taking part in any healthy eating program.

The fun part of the 16:18 diet is that you can experiment. See how your metabolism handles the change in eating habits. For some, if they confine their eating to an 8 hour window, and fast the remaining 16 hrs (including 8 hrs of sleep), they can basically eat as much as they want during those 8 hrs.

If you train yourself to simply eat until you are full (instead of overeating), you will often find it difficult to consume "too many" calories in your 8 hr window where you're allowed to eat. The secret is training your body to not "over-eat" during these periods.

By the way, one caveat to the above statement is: sugar. Consuming a lot of sugar will almost always cause you to surpass your calorie limit for the day. Natural sugars like fruit, or healthy sugars like organic dark chocolate are fine in moderation, but highly processed sugars, and sugary drinks are not your friend.

If you can manage to eat 2 big healthy filling meals a day with lots of fresh veggies and healthy fats, you will be amazed at how easy it is to shave up to 500 or 600 calories off of every single day. As this compounds and adds up, the pounds will be flying off of you.

Say if you eat a nice big lunch with avocado and cashews and some nice healthy fats that will make you feel full and satisfied. You are going to be full for quite a while. Maybe you eat a light snack at midafternoon, and then a late dinner. You won't need to consume 2500 calories--or 2000 or whatever your daily intake is--in that period of time.

Whether to choose the 5:2 or 16:8 intermittent fasting approach is very much down to the individual. 16:8, or Leangains (because it increases your lean body mass) requires the regular discipline of not eating during the 15-16 hour fast. We will get used to it very quickly, but this is a regular, daily program. Some people become bored with this approach and will begin to break it. For others, who like to plan their days in detail, then it is a perfect method to achieve weight loss.

If the diet of our choice is the 5:2 method, then we need to be the kind of person who is not going to spend our five normal days dreading the 'fasting' days. Again, remember that the word fast is an exaggeration here, on the two days we can still eat. Just not a big amount. However, if we are the kind of person who likes a bit of variety, and who would rather tough it out for 2 days instead of lightly holding back every day, then this route might be the best one for us.

Alternate Day Fasting, Including The UpDayDownDay Variation

Not eating on three or four days of the week is a challenge. It is one that requires a person with very strong will power, with the determination to see the end benefits. It is not an approach for a beginner, and as with the Eat-Stop-Eat approach (which we will look at next) the twenty-four hours is best achieved from evening meal to evening meal – going to bed hungry is not recommended.

Alternate day fasting is also not something for the beginner. Although most of us would adapt to it, trying something too extreme at the outset means we run the risk of becoming discouraged and giving up altogether. However, if we want to see quick and pleasing results, this approach delivers the goods.

A full fast for half a week (spread between normal days, remember) is probably a bit much for most people, and that is why the UpDayDownDay diet developed, created by a doctor, James Johnson. This works best for people who are disciplined and have a specific goal they want to achieve. With the best will in the world, sustaining it forever is not practical for most people (and also probably not healthy).

It operates in a very similar way to the full alternate day fasting approach but allows a small calorie intake on the down days. But the amounts are small, just 500 or so calories. In order to maximise the mix of essential nutrients needed, it is recommended to rely on meal replacement shakes on the days where eating is barred.

This is a great program for people who have the discipline to see it through and have short term goals to achieve, but it is not as sustainable as the 16:8 or 5:2 methods.

Eat-Stop-Eat

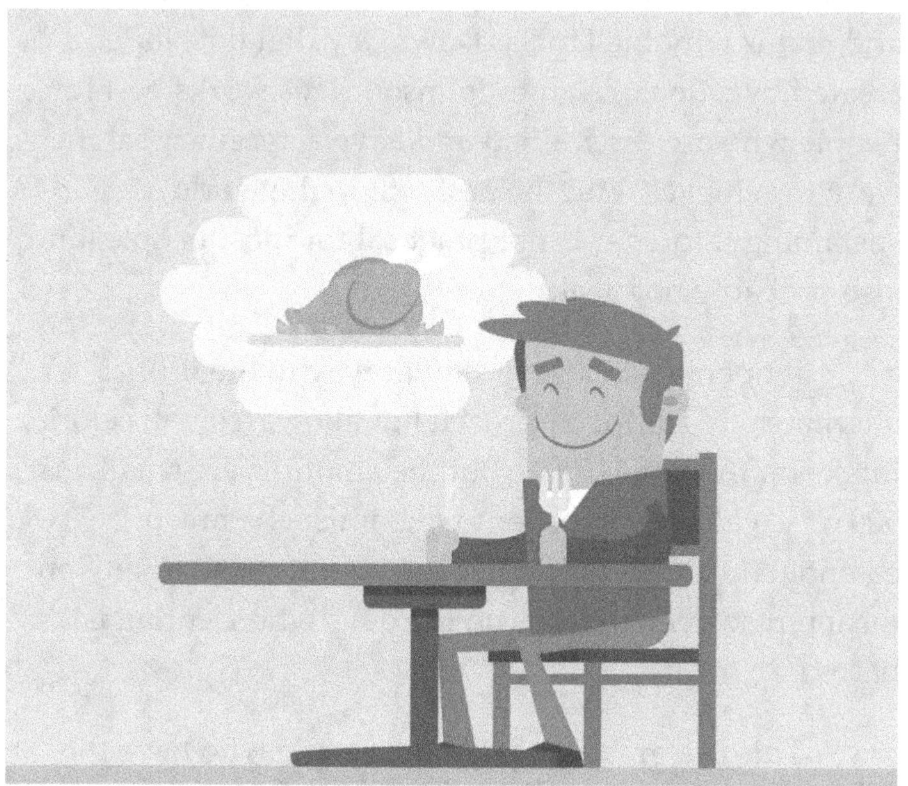

Brad Pilon, we will recall, designed this program. Basically, it requires one or two full fasting days each week. The twenty-four hours are achieved by not eating from one meal, say breakfast until the same meal the next day. This can equally be lunch to lunch, or dinner to dinner, depending on what fits best with our individual needs and wishes.

As with other fasts, it is fine (in fact, important) to drink during the food free period. This can be anything non-calorific. Drinking lots of water, for example, really helps us to feel full and to ward off any pangs of hunger.

During the non-fasting days, it is important to eat as normal, with a recommended calorie intake – a reminder that this is 2500 for men, and 2000 for women. Again, as with other diets, it is not a problem to have a slightly bigger meal after the fast.

A little warning, however: with this approach to intermittent fasting and indeed any that involve a 'full day fast' of at least twenty-four hours. The approach is perfectly safe provided we adopt a regular pattern. Our bodies will quickly adapt to a change in the way we fuel ourselves, but it gets cross if we keep changing that pattern, and the punishment it delivers is to change the way it releases hormones.

In some circumstances, hormonal imbalances can lead to illness, skin problems, mood swings and problems with sleeping. We will only have the risk of experiencing these if we keep changing our fasting pattern, so it is not a big thing to worry about as long as we are sensible.

The Eat-Stop-Eat approach does work in many ways. Our bodies will detoxify, our cells will regenerate and become healthier, we will lose weight and we will (this being the reason for the creation of the program) see our lean body mass increase while our fat stores decrease. But at a price.

Getting through a full twenty-four hour fast is a challenge. For some people, they will quickly adapt and get on well with the regime, others will find it very difficult to sustain a full day. Especially if the fast is broken by dinner. They may find it impossible not to bump up dinner by a couple of hours, or snack as the period enters its final phases. Once again, it is down to the individual – what works best for us.

If we do try this intermittent fasting program, more so than with other approaches, we need to build up gradually, with perhaps a few sixteen hour fasts before we go for the full day.

A few words for those who want to take this approach even further by planning their eating to whether they are fasting or not: Doing this will give even better results but is not for everybody. Basically, we should build the content of our eating around our exercise. Rest days should be 'fat heavy', while exercise days should be carb dominant. Exercising on fast days gives the best results.

NOTE: any type of extreme fasting diets, please make sure you consult with your doctor — it may not be advisable for everyone, particularly if you have certain types of diseases or conditions.

Warrior Diet

Another variation on the theme is the Warrior Diet, which, like many of the other approaches, was made popular by a fitness expert: Ori Hofmekler.

There are links between the Warrior Diet and other paleo diet forms, with the program requiring the consumption of raw and unprocessed vegetable and fruits.

It works like this. A four-hour eating period is allocated at night, during which we can eat as much as we like. Because, for the remainder of the day we have eaten very few calories, even a huge meal during the eating period is not going to use up a full day's worth of calories – our stomachs simply won't be able to cope with such an amount. Therefore, our overall calorie intake reduces.

Outside of this window we are allowed to consume a small quantity of raw fruits and vegetables.

The somewhat masculine name given to this approach should not put anybody off. It delivers strong results for anybody comfortable with sticking to the regime. A love of raw fruit and vegetable, and a lifestyle busy enough to occupy the long periods during the day without much in the way of food are essentials, but it is an approach that allows three food intakes during the day; and that is one of the things that helps to make it popular.

Fat Loss Forever

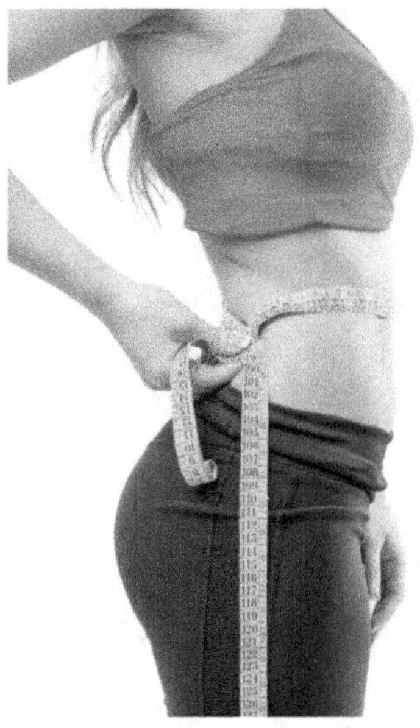

Lots of people who love dogs like to choose a mutt. The mix of genes makes these dogs less prone to illness, stronger and hardier. A mixture of the best bits of other diets can also work with intermittent fasting, as we can see with the Fat Loss Forever approach, which was developed by Dan Go and John Romaniello.

It works by taking the best bits of other diets and combining them. To add to the mix, it also throws in a bonus day…and a tough one. A cheat day exists but is followed by a full 36 hour fast, which many might find just a tad too much.

This approach is perhaps the least flexible of all, with a specific program to follow. Unlike other versions, where the fine details are down to the individual, on this diet it is important to follow the program to the letter, including the exercise program that comes with it.

For the best results, in as much as this makes the program easiest to follow, choose fasting times when you are busy, to keep the mind occupied.

It is a program that delivers strong results and works well for a short period. How sustainable it is a different question. Devotees need to have a mixture of self-discipline and a willingness to follow instructions.

If that is you, then it is worth giving this approach a try, in the short term at least.

Spontaneous Meal Skipping

There is a school of thought that believes our bodies are the best indicators of when we should eat and when we should fast. This approach is very flexible; if we do not fancy breakfast, we miss it. Not hungry at lunchtime, go without.

An approach such as this is very easy to follow but comes with some down sides. To begin with, sometimes our minds trick us – we feel virtuous by missing lunch, so have too much dinner. It is also less likely to work when the weather is cold, and we crave comfort foods.

However, keeping a diary of the meals taken should help us to keep a check on what we are eating. We do not need to include lots of details, just remember not to lose our heads over dinner or lunch, and record when we miss a meal.

There will be benefits from this approach in that our overall calorie intake drops, but because we do not enter the fasting stage, we will not get the benefits this brings. However, we can combine the two, perhaps fasting for two or three weeks, then having a spell of spontaneous meal skipping. Once again, much comes down to our individual personalities.

Here we have looked at many ways to fast intermittently; how each system operates, and how we can design our own regimes. The following key points should be remembered, though, if we are to get the benefits of weight loss plus the biological and chemical benefits of fasting.

- A spell of between 14 and 16 hours without food is needed to enter a fasting regime.

- Alternatively, we can severely limit our calorie intake for twenty-four hours to get the benefits.
- Our overall aim is to reduce calorie intake through the fasting process, so we should not binge during the non-fasting periods.

Whichever approach you finally settle on, there are some good tips to help you succeed:

- ***Set achievable, time specific goals.*** If we know where we are going, we are more likely to get there. Set milestones along the way. For example, we might aim to lose a stone in weight in three months. Set a weekly target of a pound per week and you will see yourself achieving the goal. Draw a chart of your progress, you can refer back to it in the dark times (if you have them). Once we have achieved our first goal, then set another.
- ***Drink loads of water.*** Being hydrated makes fasting easier and keeps hunger pains away.
- ***Make use of the nights.*** By fasting overnight, we are making use of dead time. It might mean missing breakfast, but that is better than going to bed hungry.
- ***Start when we are busy.*** A big vacation is not the ideal time to begin an intermittent fasting program. With less to do, our mind will drift to any hunger we are experiencing. If we are busy, then time passes more quickly, and our mind is more occupied.

- ***Exercise.*** Fasting works better with exercise, and the endorphins exercise releases will help us feel better and more positive about our fast.

Note to Consider: Cleansing Versus Lifestyle

One of the virtues of intermittent fasting, to which we return regularly, is its flexibility. We can see from the list of types of fasting that some lend themselves more fully to a lifestyle choice than others. It is hard to imagine most of us keeping up an alternate day fast for the rest of our lives; the 16:8 split is much more achievable.

However, another factor we need to consider is our goal in undertaking a program. For some, we are after the full gamut of benefits, and so need to embark on a long-term regime. For others, we seek just a short-term body cleanse. For these people, because the time spent fasting will be for only a limited period, perhaps a month or two, we can go for a harsher regime.

Chapter Summary

In this chapter we have looked at some of the ways we can undertake intermittent fasting, from some very structured approaches, to some that are much more flexible.

- We should find a system that works for us.
- There are some key points that will help us regardless of which method we choose.
- In selecting the type of intermittent fasting we choose, we should consider whether we are in it for the long haul or are seeking a short-term body cleanse.

In the next chapter we help our safety and well-being by considering some precautions to take while fasting.

Chapter Five: Intermittent Fasting Precautions

In this chapter we will learn about some of the side effects we might experience from fasting, and how to prevent or minimize them. We will also learn about the precautions we should take when embarking on our own intermittent fasting routine.

The first thing to reiterate is that for the overwhelming majority of people, fasting is a perfectly safe and very effective way to gain many benefits for our body, so the precautions and warnings ahead really need to be taken in that context. We have said, and stress again, that those with diabetes or other serious medical conditions should always take medical advice before entering into this, or any other change to their eating routine. We also stress that intermittent fasting is NOT suitable for children or the elderly, and pregnant women, or those who have recently given birth/breastfeeding.

As for everybody else, this type of diet is actually one of the safest—you are still eating a full balance of foods (for example, not severely limiting your carb intake or fats etc) and you are not taking any dangerous supplements.

One: Keep Cortisol Under Control

Cortisol is the stress hormone. When our blood sugar levels drop dramatically, which may occur when we begin our intermittent fasting, the results can be unpleasant. Cortisol makes the body produce more blood sugar to balance the drop.

When our blood sugar goes up and down quickly, a number of side effects can emerge.

- We can feel nauseous or dizzy.
- We may experience headaches.
- We become stressed. It is hard to identify what it is that is stressing us (because it is a chemical response to a physical change in this case, not a chemical response to an emotional matter), but we feel the symptoms. These include anxiety, inability to concentrate, irritability and sometimes sleep loss.

- Our moods fluctuate, which can make it difficult to stick to a routine that is new.

The way we deal with this is by not diving into a fasting regime. Just as we would train to run a half marathon, so we should train ourselves to be ready for this dietary change. The way we do this is not difficult. Before starting to fast, we ensure that, for a couple of weeks, we have eaten very well. Our diet is balanced, and regular, with lots of fruit and fiber. We eat in the morning, within a couple of hours of getting up, earlier if possible, and follow this with a lunch and dinner. We eliminate processed sugars from our diet as much possible.

This encourages our blood sugars to be strong and stable.

Dealing with our stress is more difficult. A person who is stressed has a higher level of cortisol in any case (which is a part of the reason why long-term stress can lead to other physical problems), and getting that down is harder. The best method is to exercise, eat well and get enough sleep. This will work for many, but where emotional problems are behind the stress, it can take longer to get it under control.

Diving into a fasting program could increase your stress in the short-term. Talking, perhaps even counselling can help, as can detoxing the mind by creating time for oneself through better organization, delegation and prioritization in our daily lives. Also, just as sleep and exercise are very important to stable mental health, it's also important to make time for relaxation and recreation.

Once our stress and blood sugars are under control, then the circle of benefit of intermittent dieting can really be experienced. Our weight loss and internal chemical changes help to make our blood sugar levels even better, and our stress far more readily controlled.

Two: Clearing Toxins – Unpleasant Side Effects

Fasting clears toxins from the body. This is a good thing, it makes sense that if we eliminate poisons what is left will be much healthier. However, we can experience some unpleasant short-term side effects.

- Headaches and nausea are common symptoms when detoxing, which fasting induces.

- Bad breath may be present for a short time.
- We can have stomach troubles, with short term bowel problems possible.
- We may feel tired and lethargic for a short time.

These conditions can vary from person to person and it is very possible you won't experience any of them, but careful preparation such as suggested above, plus a gradual increase in fasting times will help to reduce these symptoms or stop them from forming at all.

Three: Checking Up On Medication

Many of us take regular or occasional medication and while we may not fall into the category of "having a serious condition," it is still important to discuss with your doctor whether your fasting regime will impact your medication or if you will need to change or alter anything.

Many medications are perfectly safe with fasting; many pills actually work better when they are entering an empty stomach. Where tablets do have to be taken with food, if they are a daily dose, these can be fitted in your fasting regime, so if you are on a twenty-four hour fast, they can be taken with evening meals, when you start to eat again.

However, it is always best to check with the instructions, or with your pharmacist if you have any doubts. Always better safe than sorry.

Four: Long Lasting Symptoms

We can alleviate negative symptoms of intermittent fasting by training our bodies in preparation for the change in food intake, and by building up gradually to whatever our full intermittent fasting regime looks like. However, some of us will still experience some of the symptoms mentioned throughout this chapter.

They should disappear quickly. Anybody suffering from light-headedness, sleep problems or nausea and so on for two weeks can consider themselves unlucky. If conditions continue for more than three, then it may be that the system you are using is too extreme for your individual make up.

If so, try for an easier regime; if you are on the Warrior Diet, move to the 5:2 program. If you are fasting alternate days, or even on the Eat-Stop-Eat regime it may be that the 16:8 works better for you. If on the 16:8, try turning it into a 14:10 plan.

Listen to your body; yes, there could be short term discomfort, but it really should not be either severe, or long lasting.

Five: Extreme Fasting And Water Fasting

This topic is not really relevant to this book, but it is worth a brief mention   .

Anything longer than a couple of day's fast could result in stomach problems when we return to a normal eating pattern – it really depends on the make-up of the individual; we are also likely to feel ill, light-headed and slightly nauseous, through a long fast as our blood sugars become mixed up. Think about when we have been ill, and not eaten for a few days, the feeling of a low-level hangover is not unusual.

After five to seven days without food our electrolytes can go crazy when we start eating again; usually this will result in nausea, vomiting and diarrhea. In extreme cases, long fasts can result in serious medical problems. Any fast that is for more than forty-eight hours should always be taken only after medical advice from a suitably qualified professional.

In my opinion, water fasts should never be attempted. Dehydration can cause so many health problems both long and short term.

Chapter Summary

In this chapter we have looked at some of the side effects, and precautions, to take when starting on an intermittent fasting program. It has been a short chapter, and that is evidence of the low risk, low side effect nature of this program. Not only is it easy, cheap and effective, but also very safe.

The key points have been.

- There may be some negative side effects with intermittent fasting.
- Rarely will they last long, 2-3 weeks MAXIMUM.
- Training of the body and building up the fasting process will help to alleviate or eliminate these side effects.
- Some fasting programs, where the fasts are more than forty-eight hours, might have nastier side effects. Long term fasting can be dangerous and should only be undertaken with proper medical advice.

In the next chapter we will look a little more at the role exercise can play as we seek to gain the maximum benefits from fasting.

Chapter Six: Getting The Most Out Of Exercise

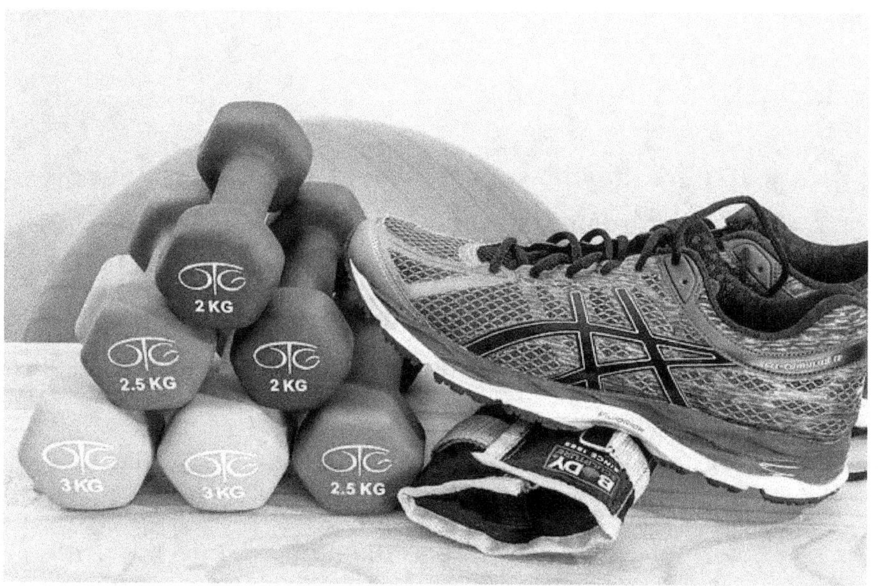

This chapter will give us an opportunity to remind ourselves of the value of exercise, and we will consider the types of exercise that are particularly beneficial to a program of intermittent fasting.

The Benefits Of Exercise

Whenever we can burn more calories than we consume, not only will we be losing weight, but we will be lowering our body fat composition. Hello sixpack! Fasting is clearly one of the best ways to keep our calorie intake low, but the best way to supercharge this and get the full range of benefits is by combining it with an exercise program.

First, for adults (ages 19-64) we are given a choice to some extent – whichever route you take, there should be a couple sessions per week to work on strength exercises to keep your muscles in shape. This is going to very much complement an intermittent fasting routine, since we know that will improve our lean body mass. On top of that should be either two and a half hours of moderate aerobic activity (which includes exercise such as cycling or walking briskly) per week, or half that amount of time in vigorous exercise. Jogging fits this category as does, for the more competitively minded, a game of singles tennis.

That minimum activity will help maintain your weight if your calorie intake is about average. It will also support our bodies as we seek to improve heart health, organ well-being and so on. So for those of us fasting, this will mean weight loss-because our calorie intake will be lower than average.

So, a brisk walk at weekends and every other day during the week is going to help us lose weight. That really is not a huge commitment. Two forty-minute trips to the gym will offer us the same benefits. However, there is one small caveat to this. While such exercise regimes as mentioned above will ensure we meet our minimum targets for good health, some daily activity is also necessary. This does not have to be severe and can be broken down into ten-minute chunks. A bit of time gardening, housework – vigorous vacuuming we might say – walking the children to school – all of these will ensure we keep sufficiently on the move.

Let us take a moment to examine the health benefits of even that minimum amount of exercise. Our chances of developing type 2 diabetes are cut in half and cut the chances of heart disease or suffering a stroke by over a third. We are more likely to live longer and some studies indicate we may reduce our chances of getting cancer by up to a half. Our bones and muscles will serve us better and for longer.

Mentally, we cut our risk of depression and of getting dementia by a third.

These benefits are all IN ADDITION TO the benefits we are already receiving from intermittent fasting (see the discussions in earlier chapters).

It is an often said — but extremely accurate — truism that our lives are increasingly sedentary. One of the best ways to get exercise is to fit it into our everyday lives. Walk instead of drive; do some strength building exercises when we get up in the morning. If we drive to work, park the car at the end of the parking lot rather than by the entrance to your office. Stroll out to a shop to get lunch or fit in a walk during your lunch break. Exercise releases endorphins, and fresh air awakens the brain – we find our afternoon performance is much improved if we have exercise during the middle of the day.

But exercise and intermittent fasting are not just two things we can do that are good for us. Most modern thinking agrees that there is a link between fasting and exercise which provides additional benefits for all the things we seek to achieve with the two activities. The sum of combining the two is greater than the individual benefits they each offer. That is synergy. With fasting and exercise combined, 2 + 2 equals 5!

We burn more calories, see better internal cell repair, see greater mental health benefits.

This is because modern thinking is challenging the age-old belief that we should not exercise on an empty stomach. When our parents told us, as children, not to swim in the sea after eating lunch, they were speaking more sense than they intended; exercise wise, a swim before lunch would have offered much better results (not that we probably needed to worry as children). What latest research is showing is that it is actually better to exercise on an empty stomach.

To conclude this section: if we exercise during our fast, the total benefit is greater than the sum of its separate parts.

Best Exercise To Enhance The Advantages Of Fasting

To get a little (but not too) scientific for a moment, the speed at which we burn fat is determined by our sympathetic nervous system (SNS). Two things stimulate our SNS – one is the exercise itself, the other is not having a stomach full of food. Thus, when we fast and exercise, we are initiating a combination of fat burning pressures. But there is more –oxidative stress increases, which promotes muscle growth and strength. Leaner. Better. Stronger.

We can fine tune this even more if we plan our exercise routines carefully.

Fasting Days: These should be used to undertake your low intensity exercise. There are two reasons for this: 1). if your sugar levels have fallen, then dizziness can strike with too much exercise, 2). if the body is desperately looking for something to burn to create energy, it may attack muscle mass, which is something we want to keep. Therefore, fasting days are great for doing walks, light swimming and gentle jogs.

Non-Fasting Days: It is therefore logical that we save our high intensity work outs for days when we have eaten. These are the times to hit the gym, to go for that long, hilly run or to rip through our laps in the pool.

Weights: If weights form part of our exercise regime, then do this on our non-fasting days. Similarly, if we are looking for high intensity short burst exercise, such as circuit training, non-fast days should be used. Also, with these types of workouts, we should eat, ideally within thirty minutes, after our exercise.

However, the joy of intermittent fasting for many people is that it is easy and flexible. For those on a serious weight loss or muscle building program, the advice above is necessary to achieve the results we seek. But for most of us, looking to get fitter, healthier and a little lighter on our feet, it is enough to remember that any exercise is good for us, no matter what form it takes.

Chapter Summary

In this chapter we have looked at exercise, and learned (or revised) the following:

- Exercise is good for us!
- In fact, exercise is essential if we are to be healthy.

- Exercising during a fast is more effective than when not fasting. That challenges traditional thinking.
- We should adapt the intensity of our exercise to our fasting program.
- But mostly, we should simply remember to do some exercise.

In the final chapter of this book we will look at some of the foods that work especially well with intermittent fasting.

Chapter Seven: What Should We Eat, And Foods To Avoid!

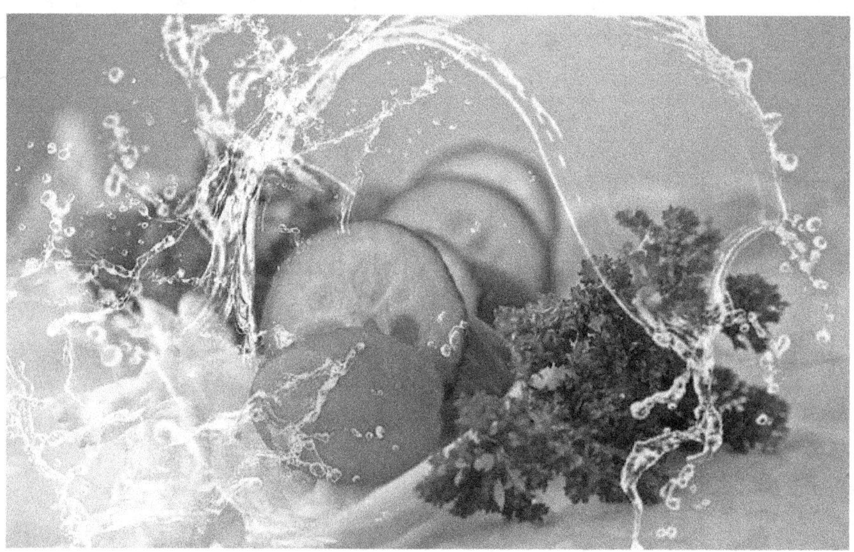

We must never make intermittent fasting difficult, because that kind of defeats the purpose. As I've already said, this dieting approach is one of the simples and most effective. In fact, many believe that part of the reason it is so effective is because of its simplicity. It is something that can fit our lifestyle, not dominate it. But, taking this into account, there are still certain food   s that will make our fasting even more effective. This chapter will take a look at this topic.

Tips For Eating On Fast Days

We are starting with a look at foods to eat on fast days, since these are more complex to work.

Of course, a lot is going to depend on how many calories you are allowing yourself on these days, but the ideas below give an insight into what is going to work well.

Foods high in protein are best for fast days. This type of food fills us up without using up too many of our calories.

Fish, chicken and eggs are perfect, as are non-animal products like tofu. These can be grilled, baked or fried with the tiniest spray of olive oil.

Vegetables top our plate and our stomachs, and can be raw, in salad form or steamed. Oven roasted with a dash of oil or boiled are other options   . It is best to avoid carbohydrates. These are high in calories and although we will feel full after eating, the sensation does not last with carbohydrates and we will soon be suffering from hunger pangs.

So you probably want to at least try to avoid pasta, rice, potatoes, and of course all processed sugars.

Sugary foods are also best avoided – honey, some fruits and vegetables such as grapes, melon, bananas and corn on the cob; it is also wise to keep away from breakfast cereals. Bread, pasta and potatoes are, of course, completely off the menu if we are seeking to keep the carbs down.

However, a bit of fat is OK. It will help us to feel full; so, although calorific in itself, it should help keep us away from other foods later in the day. Things like nuts and avocados, while high in calories, are high in very healthy fats that will make us feel full and satisfied. So these can be great to consume in moderate amounts.

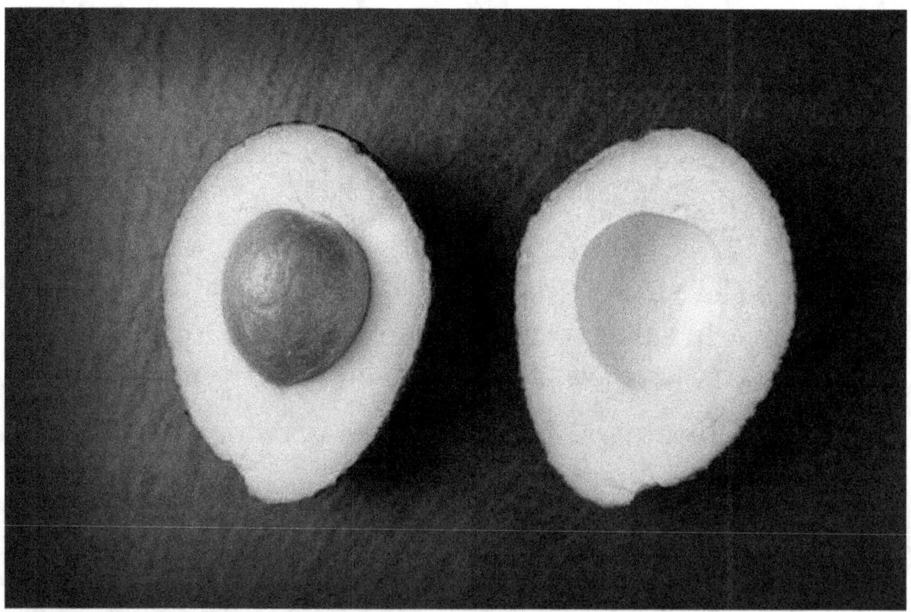

Tips For Eating On Non-Fast Days

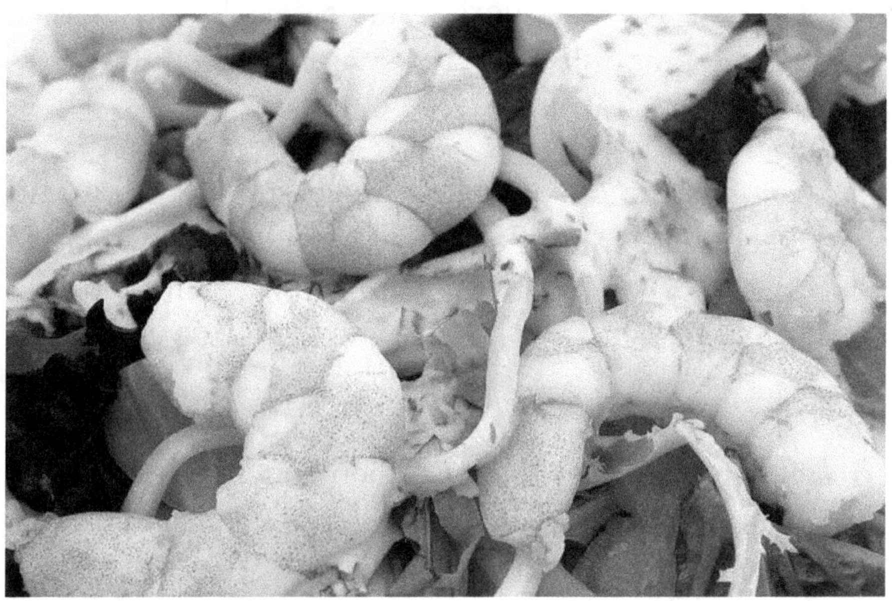

Rule 1: Eat what you like

Rule 2: in moderation

The less calories we take on board, the more weight we will lose, although we need to eat more than on our fast days because we wish to keep our body from going into starvation mode.

However, we may well find some changes after a couple of weeks in your tastes.

Firstly, as strange as it seems, we could well find ourselves less hungry than we used to be. We may not want to consume extra calories on the days following our fast. Our body may stop craving sweet, sticky stuff. We should trust what our bodies are telling us.

Another thing that we might well find is that we no longer need those mid-afternoon snacks. If we do, then it is fine to fill the gap on a non-fast day, but in all probability after a couple of weeks, those urges will disappear.

However, if they do exist, then go with them. If you are desperate for a pile of mashed potatoes on the day following your fast, then go for it. If, after six weeks or so, those urges are still present, and you find you are not losing weight, then it might be worth changing your fasting routine. We are all different, and we will each respond to different regimes.

The overall message we can offer with regards to non-fast days is, eat as our body tells us; that is likely to be pretty much in line with how we used to eat every day before starting our intermittent fasting. As long as there is no binge eating we should see the results we seek.

We should always consider our goal in deciding our eating plan. If we are after a short-term program to deliver a specific result, then we might need to stick more rigidly to the plan's suggested diet. That will mean following the fast day program as above, and keeping our calories close to, but not exceeding, recommended intakes on other days.

But if our goal is to lose weight and become healthier in the process, then it is important that our program is sustainable – there is more to life than the diet!

Nutrition

Unlike many diet plans, intermittent fasting has few nutritional risks. Because we are still eating normally during the majority of the week, we can follow the usual nutritional tips to stay healthy.

Many western diets are not particularly conducive to good health due to high levels of trans fats, refined sugars and salt. If we are to be at our optimum to get the most out of our intermittent fasting, then we need our bodies to be properly prepared, our sugar levels under control and our digestion in good order.

Nutrition is simpler than most people think. With a fasting approach, there is no need to do lots of measuring or counting and calculating nutritional values, we just need to apply common sense.

So here is a list of common sense ideas when it comes to nutrition:

- Drink plenty of fluids – water is best.
- Avoid excessive amounts of alcohol, although a glass of red wine is probably good for us (sadly, six glasses of red wine is not six times as good).
- Avoid sugary drinks. We all know about the dangers of soda and carbonated sugary drinks, but even fruit juices can be sugar heavy. Manufacturers are skilled at packaging drinks as though they are good for you, when in fact they are often not.
- Avoid excessive amounts of caffeine, but a cup or two of coffee per day is fine.
- Eat a mixture of protein, carbohydrates, fruit and vegetables.
- Eat at least five portions (which is about a handful) of fruit and vegetables a day – latest

recommendations suggest seven portions, but that's a bit ambitious.

- Natural, unprocessed foods are better than processed. So, long grain brown rice is better than white, for example.
- Include a couple of portions of fish high in omega 3 fats per week (salmon, mackerel, tuna and so forth).
- Limit fried food as it is highly saturated in fat making it extremely caloric while having very little nutritive value.
- Use vegetable oils such as olive rather than other fats to cook with.

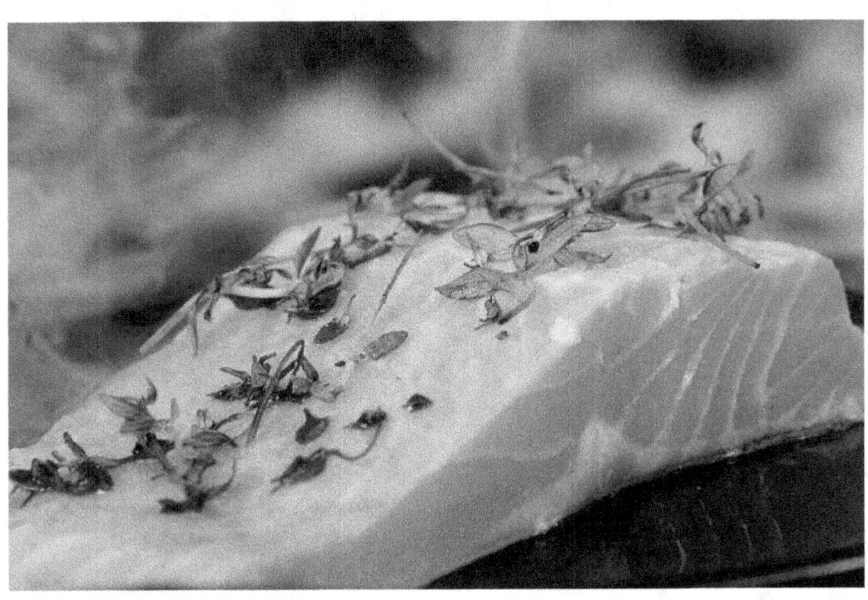

Following this kind of nutritional advice will help to keep our bodies fit. But remember, while intermittent fasting can produce quick results, the most sustainable diets are the ones that occur over time. And to achieve long term results, the diet must fit to our life, not our life to the diet.

Chapter Summary

In this, our final chapter we have looked at the food types that fit well with this form of diet.

- Normal eating habits on non-fast days, and reduced on fast days works well
- It's simple
- High protein works well on fast days.
- Simply achieving a good nutritional balance is all that is needed to maintain good health; there is no need to undertake complex recipes or remove food groups from our diet. Although, equally, if for example, a ketogenic diet is what you fancy, then go for it.

Final Words

Many thanks for buying this book. I hope that it has helped your understanding of the world of intermittent fasting. We hope that it has encouraged you to try this easy, cheap and highly effective way of improving health and waist line with really very little pain.

As we finish, we will summarize the main points of our tome.

We should properly start with safety. Please remember that while fasting is suitable for nearly everybody except for those mentioned in earlier sections of this book, it's still always a good idea to consult with your doctor before making any big diet changes.

For most, it is a great way to get health and weight-loss benefits. Most medications are fine with intermittent fasting, but check the notes that come with your pills, and seek advice from your pharmacist if you have any doubts.

Intermittent fasting, we have learned, is a general term that is put into practice in many ways. It simply involves having periods when we eat very little or not at all.

Generally, our bodies and minds get used to any changes in our eating habits in two or three weeks, but sometimes it can take longer. With so many flexible ways to employ this weight control method, we may need to try a few different methods to find what works best for us. It is always a good idea to build up to our fasting regime by starting with smaller periods of fast, and spending some time getting ourselves into the habit of eating a good diet.

Long term fasting is a different matter and could lead to health problems. Medical advice should be taken before embarking on any fast that goes beyond a couple of days.

On the other hand, intermittent fasting is likely to allow us to gain many medical benefits. Included here are protection against diabetes, heart disease, cancers and strokes. Blood pressure and blood sugars will improve, our digestion will get better and mentally our well-being is likely to improve. We may even protect ourselves against Alzheimer's and Parkinson's disease.

We are even likely to develop appetite control. All of this can be achieved without any special diet beyond what our bodies tell us and a touch of common sense, and in a way, that allows us to sustain the fasting within our desired lifestyle.

Intermittent fasting really is a superb way to lose weight and improve our health; I urge you to make it a part of your life.

About the Author:

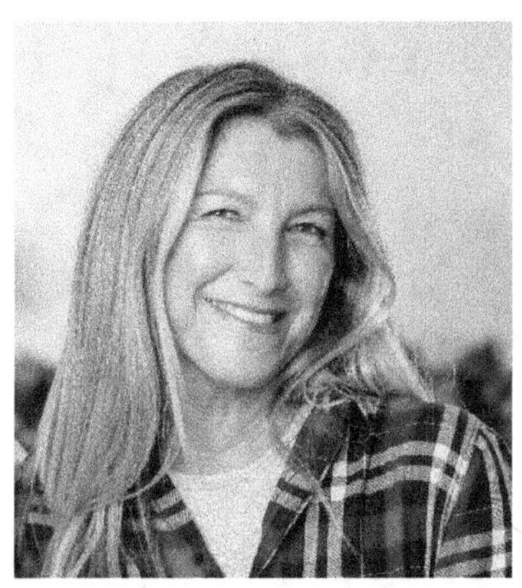

Linda Becker is an entrepreneur, yoga instructor, author, and proud mother of 3. She runs a successful chain of yoga studios with branches across the country. After helping many of her yoga clients achieve incredible results with her intermittent dieting plans, she was inspired to write this book to help others achieve the same results. She lives in Wisconsin with her husband and children.